Emerg
Echocardiography

D1758102

Emergency Echocardiography

Adrian Chenzbraun MD, FESC

Consultant Cardiologist, Clinical Lead, Echocardiography
The Royal Liverpool University Hospital
The Liverpool Heart and Chest Hospital
Liverpool, UK

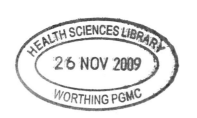

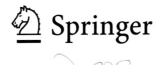 Springer

2009

Adrian Chenzbraun
The Royal Liverpool University Hospital
Liverpool, UK

The correct eISBN is 978-1-84882-336-5.

DOI: 10.1007/978-1-84882-336-5_14

ISBN 978-1-84882-335-8   e-ISBN 978-1-84800-336-5
DOI: 10.1007/978-1-84882-336-5

British Library Cataloguing in Publication Data

Library of Congress Control Number: 2008942043

© Springer-Verlag London Limited 2009
Apart from any fair dealing for the purposes of research or private study,
or criticism or review, as permitted under the Copyright, Designs and
Patents Act 1988, this publication may only be reproduced, stored or
transmitted, in any form or by any means, with the prior permission in
writing of the publishers, or in the case of reprographic reproduction in
accordance with the terms of licences issued by the Copyright Licensing
Agency. Enquiries concerning reproduction outside those terms should be
sent to the publishers.
The use of registered names, trademarks, etc. in this publication does not
imply, even in the absence of a specific statement, that such names are
exempt from the relevant laws and regulations and therefore free for general
use.
Product liability: The publisher can give no guarantee for information
about drug dosage and application thereof contained in this book. In every
individual case the respective user must check its accuracy by consulting
other pharmaceutical literature.

Printed on acid-free paper

Springer is part of Springer Science + Business Media (www.springer.com)

Foreword

Echocardiography has certainly become the mostly used non-invasive imaging technology in the assessment of cardiac function. Several technical refinements over the years have made it a superb diagnostic tool in different clinical settings, including the intensive (ICU, intensive care unit)/emergency (ER, emergency room) care atmosphere. The ability to perform transesophageal studies, to use contrast or three dimensional echo and fully assess the hemodynamics at bedside in a reliable way, or use a hand-held device, among others, has added significant value and accuracy to the way patients are currently managed in the ICU/ER. It is also a reality that echocardiography has expanded beyond the boundaries of cardiology, which is unavoidable (and maybe even desirable). It is, however, important to strongly underline the need of proper knowledge and training in order to make it a useful and reliable method. This encompasses a whole set of different approaches, including practical training and adequate sources of information and study. This book by Adrian Chenzbraun certainly fulfils this goal in several ways. In opposition to the conventional classical books, sometimes with too many theoretical details that make the reader a bit lost, in this book there was great care in making it a useful bedside tool with very practical tips, profuse illustrations demonstrating the main uses, pitfalls, and tricks of echocardiography in the emergency setting. With great wit the author provides very practical algorithms for the different clinical situations. Consequently, this is a book not only for the ones who are starting to use the technique but also will certainly be a great help for the experienced echocardiologist or intensivist. Certainly, the extensive experience of the author in the field helped in crafting this book and turning it into a real practical advisor.

I will finish with a quote 2,400 years old from Hippocrates, which I think applies perfectly to this book: "Everyone has a doctor in him or her; we just have to help it in its work." *Emergency Echocardiography* will certainly be a great help for all of those who will use it for their clinical work.

Fausto J. Pinto
Professor of Cardiology, Lisbon University, Portugal
Past President of European Association of Echocardiography (EAE)
Lisbon, September 25, 2008

Preface

The idea of writing this book arose from frequent encounters with cardiologists in training and intensivist colleagues who highlighted the contribution of echocardiographic studies to the evaluation of difficult cases. In this, our experience only mirrored the growing role of echocardiography in the immediate management of hemodynamically unstable or acutely ill patients, as increasingly acknowledged in the literature.[1-3]

Echocardiography is the most versatile cardiac imaging technology readily available today at the patient's bedside. Its superb diagnostic input relates to the ability to identify any hemodynamic condition and cardiac pathology that implies a morphologic and/or a flow pattern change. Impressive technological advances over the last half century (Table I.1) and the advent of small, portable, and yet powerful echocardiographic machines pushed this technique in the frontline of diagnostic strategies when dealing with critically ill patients. Indeed, we are witnessing a change of medical practice, whereby, the management of hemodynamically unstable patients relies less on invasive data and increasingly more on the noninvasive assessment immediately obtainable with echocardiography.

It is the aim of this book to be a step-by-step, *how-* and *what-to-do*, easy to use guide for the benefit of cardiology and intensive care doctors and sonographers faced with critically ill patients for whom major therapeutic decisions could depend on the information provided by a timely and accurate echocardiographic examination. It tries to address what was perceived to be the practical needs of cardiology trainees and of intensivists faced with the increased use of echocardiography in an acute care setting. Because of the intended dual audience of this book, both pure "cardiological" topics such as aortic pathology, valvular emergencies, mechanical complications of myocardial infarction, or tamponade and more "intensive care" or "mixed" situations such as pulmonary embolism, resuscitation, sepsis, and the need for filling status assessment are covered.

Table I.1   Echocardiographical historical landmarks

Year	Development	
1954	First M-mode study	
1970s	2D technology	
1980s	Spectral and color Doppler	
1990s and 2000s	<u>Techniques</u>	<u>Technologies</u>
	TEE	3D echocardiography
	Stress echocardiography	Second harmonic and
	Intraoperative	contrast echocardiography
	echocardiography	Tissue Doppler echocardi-
	Intravascular	ography
	echocardiography	
	Intracardiac	
	echocardiography	
	Hand-held	
	echocardiography	

2D two-dimensional, *3D* three-dimensional, *TEE* transesophageal echocardiography

The users of this guide should have an echocardiography expertise roughly equivalent to at least level 1, that is, able to understand echocardiographic studies and information and ideally level 2.[4] A special case, however, is that of acute and intensive care doctors for whom a more basic and targeted understanding of echocardiographic practice may be adequate to address a few major and well-defined pathologies in a focused way.[5]

The book starts with an opening chapter dedicated to the essentials of echocardiographic technology, standard imaging, newer techniques and practical, and "don't forget to ..." tips to perform a study with diagnostic value. Evolving technologies which are yet to be adopted into routine clinical practice such as three-dimensional echocardiography or speckle tracking are not discussed. Beginning with fundamental concepts and then reviewing the main controls and settings of an echocardiographic machine, this section was written having in mind the less-experienced echocardiographer, possibly not a cardiologist, who nevertheless may have to perform an urgent study at a time when no one more skilled is available for help and advice. However, this chapter addresses the basic concepts only and, thus, is to be seen as an aid, and in no way as a substitute for a proper training in performing a basic echocardiographic examination. Also, any information or guideline provided by this book should be individualized and selectively applied in a given case, using clinical judgment and the advice of a more experienced colleague, if needed.

The various applications of echocardiography in critically ill patients are discussed in the following sections, trying to strike the right balance between a didactic approach and a practical one; whereby, a clinical scenario is used to raise the questions which should be answered by an echocardiographic study. More specialized topics and practical issues are summarized in appendixes to be found at the end of the book. Essential indexed references are provided at the end of each chapter and they are supplemented by a list of general references and resources in Appendix H.

Unless mentioned otherwise, all figures are from the author's personal collection.

The possible mentioning or identification of echocardiographic equipment throughout the text should in no way be seen as an endorsement of the particular brand involved.

References

1. Vieillard-Baron A, Slama M, Cholley B, Janvier G, Vignon P. Echocardiography in the intensive care unit: from evolution to revolution? *Intensive Care Med.* 2008;34(2):243–249.
2. Vieillard-Baron A, Prin S, Chergui K, Dubourg O, Jardin F. Hemodynamic instability in sepsis: bedside assessment by Doppler echocardiography. *Am J Respir Crit Care Med.* 2003;168(11):1270–1276.
3. Kendall JL, Hoffenberg SR, Smith RS. History of emergency and critical care ultrasound: the evolution of a new imaging paradigm. *Crit Care Med.* 2007;35(Suppl. 5):S126–S130.
4. Quinones MA, Quinones MA, Douglas PS, Foster E et al. ACC/AHA clinical competence statement on echocardiography: A Report of the American College of Cardiology/American Heart Association/American College of Physicians-American Society of Internal Medicine Task Force on Clinical Competence Developed in Collaboration with the American Society of Echocardiography, the Society of Cardiovascular Anesthesiologists, and the Society of Pediatric Echocardiography. *J Am Coll Cardiol.* 2003; 41:687–708.
5. Beaulieu Y. Specific skill set and goals of focused echocardiography for critical care clinicians. *Crit Care Med.* 2007;35(Suppl. 5):S144–S149.

Acknowledgments

This book would not have been possible without the hard work and support of sonographers at the Royal Liverpool University Hospital and the Liverpool Heart and Chest Hospital.

Special thanks to friends and colleagues who reviewed the manuscript and whose suggestions have been incorporated in the final text.

About the Author

Dr. Adrian Chenzbraun was trained in echocardiography at Stanford University, CA. He has authored numerous articles in peer-reviewed medical journals. Presently, he is a consultant cardiologist and clinical lead in echocardiography at the Royal Liverpool University Hospital and the Liverpool Heart and Chest Hospital.

Contents

Symbols and Abbreviations

2D	two dimensional
3D	three dimensional
ACS	acute coronary syndrome
AD	aortic dissection
AF	atrial fibrillation
AMI	acute myocardial infarction
AML	anterior mitral leaflet
AO	aorta
APM	anterolateral papillary muscle
AR	aortic regurgitation
AS	aortic stenosis
ASD	atrial septal defect
AV	aortic valve
AVA	aortic valve area
AVR	aortic valve replacement
AVSR	acute ventricular septal rupture
BP	blood pressure
CAUSE	Cardiac Arrest Ultrasound Examination
CBV	central blood volume
CE	contrast echocardiography
CMP	cardiomyopathy
COLD	chronic obstructive lung disease
CPR	cardiopulmonary resuscitation
CRT	cardiac resynchronization therapy
CSA	cross-sectional area
CT	computed tomography
CVP	central venous pressure
CW	continuous wave
DA	descending aorta
DT	deceleration time
EDV	end-diastolic volume
EGALS	Echo Guided Advanced Life Support
EMEA	European Medicines Agency
EROA	effective regurgitant orifice area

ESV	end-systolic volume
FAST	Focused Assessment by Sonography in Trauma
FDA	Food and Drugs Administration
FEER	Focused Echocardiographic Evaluation in Resuscitation
FL	false lumen
FPS	frames per second
HCU	hand-carried ultrasound
IABP	intraaortic balloon pump
IAS	interatrial septum
IE	infective endocarditis
IMET	Immediate Echocardiographic Triage
IMH	intramural hematoma
IP	intrapericardial pressure
ICU	intensive care unit
IVC	inferior vena cava
IVS	interventricular septum
LA	left atrium
LAA	left atrial appendage
LAD	left anterior descending coronary artery
LBBB	left bundle branch block
LCA	left carotid artery
LCC	left coronary cusp
LCx	left circumflex coronary artery
LMCA	left main coronary artery
LSA	left subclavian artery
LUPV	left upper pulmonary vein
LV	left ventricle
LVAD	left ventricular assist device
LVAW	left ventricle anterior wall
LVEDP	left ventricular end-diastolic pressure
LVEF	left ventricular ejection fraction
LVIW	left ventricle inferior wall
LVLW	left ventricular lateral wall
LVO	left ventricle opacification
LVOT	left ventricle outflow tract
LVPW	left ventricular posterior wall
LVT	left ventricular thrombus
MI	myocardial infarction
MPA	main pulmonary artery
MR	mitral regurgitation
MRI	magnetic resonance imaging
MS	mitral stenosis
MV	mitral valve

MVA	mitral valve area
NCC	non-coronary cusp
$P_{1/2}T$	pressure half-time
PAP	pulmonary artery pressure
PCI	percutaneous coronary intervention
PCWP	pulmonary capillary-wedged pressure
PDA	posterior descending artery
PE	pulmonary embolism
PEA	pulseless electrical activity
PF	pericardial fluid
PFO	patent foramen ovale
PHT	pulmonary hypertension
PISA	proximal isovelocity surface area
PML	posterior mitral leaflet
PPM	posteromedial papillary muscle
PSLA	parasternal long axis
PSSA	parasternal short-axis view
PV	pulmonic valve
PW	pulsed wave
RA	right atrium
RAA	right atrial appendage
RAP	right atrial pressure
RCA	right coronary artery
RCC	right coronary cusp
RF	regurgitant fraction
RPA	right pulmonary artery
RV	right ventricle
RVOT	right ventricle outflow tract
RVSP	right ventricular systolic pressure
SAM	systolic anterior motion
SBP	systolic blood pressure
SPW	subxyphoid pericardial window
SV	stroke volume
SVC	superior vena cava
TC	Takotsubo cardiomyopathy
TD	tissue Doppler
TEE	transesophageal echocardiography
TGC	time gain controls
TIA	transient ischemic attack
TL	true lumen
TR	tricuspid regurgitation
TTE	transthoracic echocardiography
TV	tricuspid valve

US	ultrasound
VC	vena contracta
VF	ventricular fibrillation
VSD	ventricular septal defect
VTI	velocity time integral

Chapter 1
Getting Ready for the Study

The amount and complexity of possible controls of an echocardiographic machine and the involved physical principles can be bewildering without full technical training. This chapter deals with basic theoretical assumptions and the mastering of those controls, which are necessary to perform a clinically useful study. Suggestions for controls optimization are provided in a practical manner, as well as tips to avoid frequent artifacts. Increasingly popular techniques, such as tissue Doppler and contrast echocardiography, are explained with an emphasis on practical aspects of their use. All standard echocardiographic views are presented, using a rich iconography, and highlighting the potential clinical information provided.

1.1 ULTRASOUND SYSTEMS BASICS

From the simplest to the most sophisticated, any echocardiography system will consist of the following basic components:

- Transducer(s)
- Computing system to process the ultrasound signal
- Screen display
- Analogic (VCR tape recorder) and/or digital (optical disk/DVD) storage capacity

Among the numerous technical parameters and concepts related to the use of ultrasound for medical diagnostic purposes, the following represents a minimum to be fully understood even

A. Chenzbraun, *Emergency Echocardiography*, DOI: 10.1007/978-1-84882-336-5_1,
© Springer-Verlag London Limited 2009

by "occasional" users, if they are to obtain a diagnostic quality study. For more in-depth presentation of the physics of ultrasound imaging, the reader is referred to available general echocardiography textbooks (Appendix H).

1.2 ULTRASOUND FREQUENCY AND WAVELENGTH (FIG. 1.1)

By definition, ultrasound has a frequency above 20,000 Hz, which is the upper limit of the audible spectrum of the human ear. The usual range of frequencies for cardiology diagnostic purposes is much higher: 1.5–5.0 MHz for transthoracic (TTE) studies, 5–7 MHz for transesophageal studies, and 7–10 MHz for intracardiac studies. As opposed to first-generation mechanical transducers, present phased array ones have a small footprint so they can be used even with a narrow intercostal space and are able to deliver several frequencies, which can be selected with the appropriate controls.

The actual frequency is displayed along with other technical data on the machine screen (Fig. 1.2). For a given propagation velocity (around 1,500 m/s in soft tissues), these high frequencies ensure wavelengths <1 mm, which are suitable for the visualizations of cardiac structures. The concept of wavelength is important since it defines image resolution (see below).

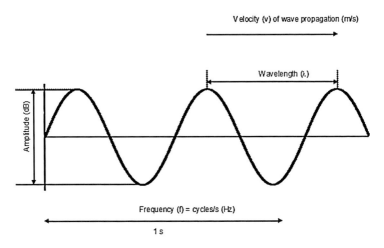

FIG. 1.1. Schematic representation of an ultrasound wave.

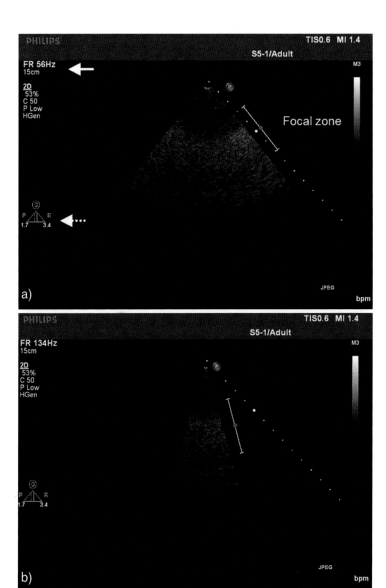

Fɪɢ. 1.2. Screen snapshot (*in this example a Philips IE 33 machine*) displaying main settings and imaging characteristics. The transducer frequencies in harmonic imaging are displayed on the left side with a triangle symbol (*dotted arrow*); the lower number is the emitted frequency and the higher one, the received harmonic frequency. The frame rate (Hz) and the image depth (cm) are displayed in the left upper corner (*thick arrow*). *A thin line with a central dot* shows the position of the focal zone, where ultrasound energy is maximal. **a** Large sector width. **b** Narrow sector width. Note the increase in frame rate from 56 Hz to 134 Hz when using a narrow sector.

1.3 INTERACTION OF ULTRASOUND WITH TISSUES AND IMAGE FORMATION (FIG. 1.3)

1.3.1 Reflection

The ultrasound image is generated when the main ultrasound beam is reflected by the targeted structure and thus redirected toward the transducer. Reflection occurs at interfaces between media of different acoustic impedance, that is, with different densities and ultrasound propagation velocities. When the differences in impedance are high, such as for pericard, bone, air, heavily calcified structures, or prosthetic material, the intensity of the reflected signal is high as well, while the blood-myocardium interface is a much weaker reflector and will return a small amount of the incident signal. Strong reflectors may totally block the ultrasound signal distal to them (the so-called "shadowing" noted with prosthetic valves) or induce artifacts whereby the ultrasound signal "travels" back and forth between the transducer and an anatomical structure.

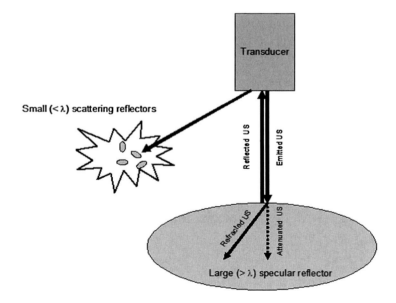

FIG. 1.3. Schematic representation of ultrasound interaction with targets of different sizes (See text for details).

1.3.2 Scattering

For the kind of directional, "mirror-like" reflection described above to occur, the target has to have a lateral dimension greater than the ultrasound wavelength (specular reflector). If the target dimensions are smaller than the ultrasound wavelength, it will behave as a scattering reflector and the ultrasound will be redirected in all directions. Scattering is not suitable for morphological imaging as needed in two-dimensional (2D) echocardiography but is used in Doppler echocardiography and tissue characterization techniques.

1.3.3 Refraction

Part of the ultrasound beam changes its direction at the interface between media of different acoustic impedance in the same way as light rays change their path when they pass through a lens. Occasionally, this phenomenon can induce artifacts as well.

1.3.4 Attenuation

Loss of energy (attenuation) occurs while the ultrasound travels through the tissue, limiting the distance at which a target can be effectively interrogated. The loss of energy increases at higher frequencies, so a loss in penetration is the price to be paid when high frequencies are used to improve resolution (see below). Attenuation occurs in fact twice, once when the transmitted ultrasound penetrates the tissue and again, on its way back from the reflecting target to the transducer. As a result, ultrasound signals from targets remote from the transducer are extremely weak and need a preferential amplification. This is achieved through the time-gain-compensation controls, which allow for the signals returning later (thus, coming from a greater distance) to be selectively amplified.

1.3.5 Image Resolution

Represents the minimal distance at which two discrete targets are still seen as separate. In practical terms, a higher resolution means a more detailed image of a given structure. 2D resolution is better along the ultrasound beam (axial resolution) than on its sides (lateral resolution). With higher frequencies, resolution increases (up to 1 mm); however, ultrasound penetration decreases.

- High frequencies should be tried in children, youngsters, and thin-chested individuals where loss of penetration is of less concern.
- Low frequencies offer less quality but may allow reasonable imaging in elderly, overweight, thick-chest patients.
- Focusing on the area of interest and reducing the transmitted power (mechanical index) may improve lateral resolution.

1.3.6 Frame Rate

Not to be confused with frequency, the frame rate, expressed in frames per second (fps) or Hz, shows how many times per second the image renews itself. High rates will provide a smooth image while low rates will not only be "jerky" but may also miss short-lived events, especially in tachycardic patients. Modern systems should allow 2D imaging at frame rates above 30 fps. Tissue Doppler (TD) imaging on the other side requires much higher (>100 fps) frame rates. The actual frame rate is displayed on the machine screen for information purposes (Fig. 1.2) and, in some high-end machines, it can be directly controlled. The available frame rate will reflect a balance between the quality of the transducer, the computing power of the system, and the size and complexity of the scan as determined by other parameters.

To increase frame rate:

- Reduce depth-of-field
- Narrow sector width
- Avoid simultaneous spectral and color Doppler imaging
- When in color mode, use the B/W suppress function

1.3.7 Mechanical Index

Ultrasound amplitude is expressed in decibels (dB) and its intensity is measured in watt/cm^2. The mechanical index is used to quantify the mechanical effects. It is a dimensionless parameter, defined as the ratio of the maximal negative pressure to the square root of the frequency. Medical diagnostic ultrasound systems are required to use a mechanical index <1.9 to avoid cavitation, that is, rapid formation and destruction of gas bubbles.[1] The usual mechanical index for a standard echocardiographic study is about 1.4 but much lower values are used for contrast studies.

1.4 FUNDAMENTAL AND SECOND HARMONIC IMAGING

The propagation of the ultrasound waves through the target tissues generates secondary ultrasound waves with frequencies which are multiples of the transmitted (fundamental) ultrasound. In fundamental imaging, the reflected harmonic frequencies ultrasound is filtered out and only the fundamental one is processed to generate the echo image. If an opposite algorithm is used whereby the reflected fundamental frequency ultrasound is filtered out and the second harmonic one is processed to generate the echo image, the modality is called harmonic imaging. Since harmonic signals are generated at a higher depth of field, they will be less distorted by obstacles close to the transducer, such as bony structures. The provided resolution will also be better due to higher frequencies. Initially targeted for use with contrast echocardiography, second harmonic imaging was found useful without contrast as well to improve image quality and became the standard for 2D imaging. The actual modality, that is, fundamental or harmonic is displayed on the machine screen (Fig. 1.2). The potential drawback used to be some artifactual brightening and thickening of the anatomic structures though this is of less concern with modern machines.

- Use second harmonic imaging either as routine or whenever the image quality is unsatisfactory.
- Beware of possible increased tissue brightness seen with this modality.
  - Some typical patterns such as the ground-glass or sparkling appearance of cardiac amyloidosis have been described using fundamental imaging.
  - If in doubt, double-check with fundamental imaging.

1.5   BLOOD FLOW DOPPLER IMAGING

This technique applies the Doppler principle whereby the difference between the frequency of the emitted ultrasound and that of the ultrasound scattered by the moving red blood cells is used to compute both the velocity and direction of the blood flow (Appendix A). Flow Doppler imaging is utilized to analyze regurgitant and stenotic flows. There are two flow Doppler imaging modalities: spectral and color Doppler.

1.5.1   Spectral Doppler (Fig. 1.4)

The display is a waveform showing the direction and velocity of the blood in an area of interest. Its main uses are to determine velocities and gradients. Spectral Doppler can be used as either pulsed wave (PW) when the same transducer alternatively acts as an ultrasound emitter and receiver or as continuous wave (CW) Doppler when two transducers act simultaneously, one as emitter and one as receiver. The former allows interrogation of a distinct area of interest (i.e., a stenotic valve) but can be used up to a certain velocity only (Nyquist limit), beyond which the signal becomes turbulent. The latter allows accurate display of high velocities but cannot reliably locate the site of flow acceleration.

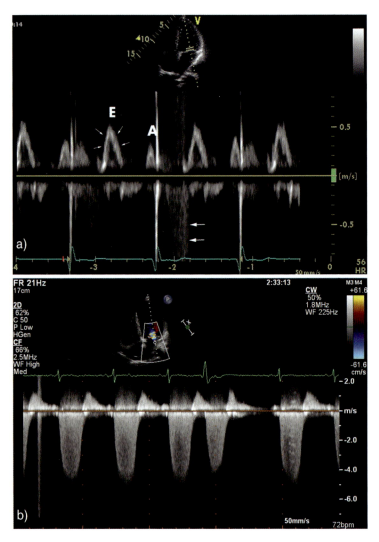

FIG. 1.4. Spectral Doppler display. **a** Pulsed wave (*PW*) imaging of a normal mitral inflow with the rapid filling (E) and atrial filling (A) components. The flow is laminar and the low velocities are fully displayed and uniformly distributed within a narrow envelope (*thin arrows*). The systole is filled by the flow of existent mitral regurgitation (*thick arrows*), which due to high velocities cannot be resolved by the PW mode and is aliasing above and below the isoelectric line. **b** Continuous wave (*CW*) imaging of a high velocity, turbulent mitral regurgitation flow. In this case, color display was used for optimal positioning of the CW line within an eccentric jet. Note

- Use PW to assess low velocity flow patterns and to pinpoint the site of flow acceleration.
- Use CW to display high velocity flows.

1.5.2 Color Doppler (Fig. 1.5)

This is essentially a PW modality where color-coded pixels are displayed instead of a waveform, whenever blood motion is detected. By convention, red encodes flow toward the transducer and blue encodes flow away from the transducer. Since Nyquist limit applies,

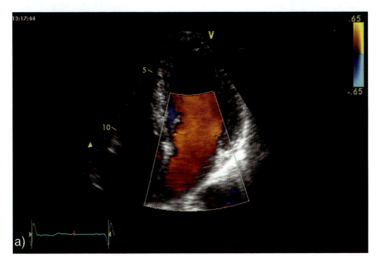

FIG. 1.5. Color Doppler imaging. **a** Transmitral normal diastolic flow. *The smooth red color* indicates laminar, low velocity flow below the upper limit of the color Nyquist scale in the right upper part of the image. **b** Transmitral systolic flow in a case of severe mitral regurgitation. The color display gives an overall image of the flow distribution and the mosaic appearance reflects the high velocity, turbulent jet. The Nyquist limits are –65 cm/s to +65 cm/s in the *panel (a)* and –51 cm/s to +51 cm/s in the *panel (b)*.

FIG. 1.4. (continued) that the systolic velocities are filling the whole signal spectrum, indicating the high variance typical of a turbulent jet. The high velocity flow is fully resolved by the CW mode, without aliasing. The scale (–0.8 m/s to +0.8 m/s in the upper panel and –7 m/s to +2 m/s in the lower panel) and the position of the 0 line should be adjusted for optimal display to accommodate the velocities recorded.

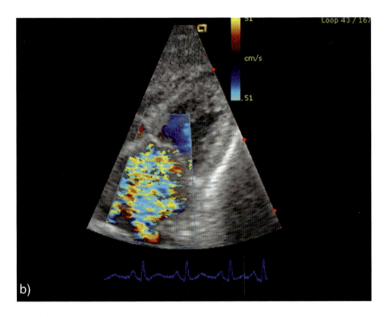

Fig. 1.5. (continued)

high velocity turbulent flows appear as a mosaic of colors. Color Doppler is used to visually map abnormal flows and provides a generally reliable assessment of their location and extent.

1.6 TISSUE DOPPLER (TD) IMAGING

Using a different filtering algorithm, the same physical principle as in flow Doppler is applied to the higher amplitude, lower velocity signals generated by cardiac walls motion during the cardiac cycle, allowing for the analysis of both systolic and diastolic events. As for flow Doppler, TD can be used as a color map superimposed over the 2D image (Fig. 1.6) or as a spectral PW modality to provide a waveform display of the direction and velocity of wall motion (Fig. 1.7). The color mapping can be used at a later time for offline analysis with the help of dedicated software while PW TD provides online velocity readings at the time of the study. The waveforms obtained by the two modalities are similar, though the velocities readings with software analysis of the color map are lower than those measured directly with PW. TD is used mainly to characterize systolic and diastolic function and to guide cardiac resynchronization therapy with biventricular pacing.

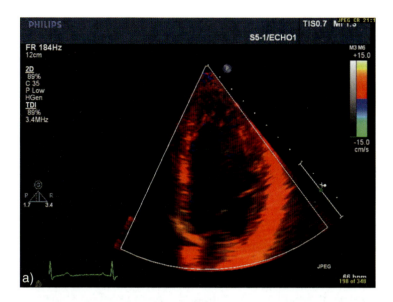

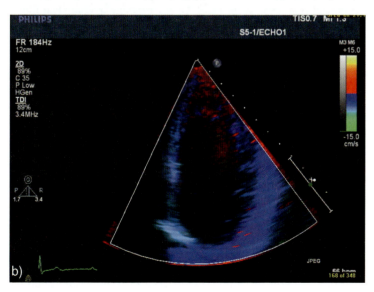

FIG. 1.6. Color tissue Doppler map superimposed over a two-dimensional image in apical 4-chamber view of a patient with normal systolic function. **a** Systolic frame: all segments are red-encoded, showing motion toward the apex. **b** Diastolic frame: all segments are blue-encoded, showing motion away from the apex.

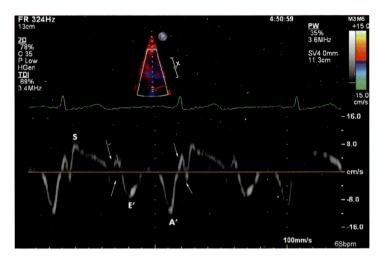

Fig. 1.7. Typical pulsed wave tissue Doppler tracing. The sample volume is placed at the septal aspect of the mitral annulus. In systole, the mitral valve plane moves toward the apex, producing a positive wave (S). In diastole, the motion is in the opposite direction and mirrors the ventricular filling phases as displayed in flow Doppler echocardiography. *S*: systolic wave, *E'*: early diastolic wave, *A'*: atrial diastolic wave. The biphasic components before and after the S wave represent the isovolumic contraction and relaxation phases (*arrows*).

1.7 CONTRAST ECHOCARDIOGRAPHY WITH TRANSPULMONARY AGENTS

Even with modern transducers, 10–30% of patients will have suboptimal images,[2,3] resulting in limited left ventricle (LV) visualization and inaccurate contractility assessment. Contrast echocardiography with left ventricle opacification (LVO) fills the LV cavity with strong echoes, while the myocardium remains black and allows a good delineation of the blood-endocardial border. The motion of LV segments and the degree of systolic thickening are thus well visualized providing a superior qualitative assessment of ventricular contractility and a more reliable calculation of ejection fraction with less interobserver variability. Several echo contrast agents are available (Table 1.1), with different chemical composition and physical properties but all have as common denominator a small size (3–5 μm, i.e., similar to the erythrocytes size) of the echogenic microspheres. This allows them to pass through the pulmonary circulation and reach the left heart after a peripheral vein administration. The microspheres resonate when exposed to the ultrasound waves and generate strong echo signals, providing a good endocardial-blood demarcation even in difficult subjects (Fig. 1.8).

Imaging with contrast agents requires a low mechanical index of 0.3–0.7 (as opposed to 1–1.5 during usual examination) to avoid quick destruction of the microspheres. This can be achieved either

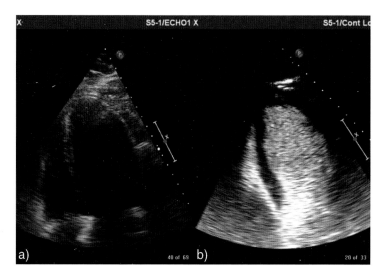

FIG. 1.8. Side-by-side comparison of images obtained in an apical 4-chamber view in a patient with a poor apical acoustic window. **a** Second harmonic imaging without contrast. Note poor delineation of the basal septum and lateral wall segments and the near-field artifacts in the apical area. **b** Contrast used with a left ventricular opacification protocol. There is excellent demarcation of the blood-endocardium interface allowing good quantification of left ventricle size and function.

TABLE 1.1. Commonly available contrast agents for echocardiography.

Generation	Manufacturer	Name	Type (microsphere wall/contained gas)
1	Malinckrodt	Albunex	Albumin/air
1	Schering	Levovist	Lipid/air
2	Malinckrodt	Optison	Albumin/perfluoropropane
2	Bracco	SonoVue	Phospholipid/sulphur hexafluoride
2	DuPont	Definity	Liposome/perfluoropropane

manually, by lowering the MI, or by using the machine built-in setup for contrast studies. The contrast agent is prepared following the manufacturer's instructions and, generally, given as a bolus through an antecubital vein using a cannula with a   20G lumen and avoiding valved ports or side arms. The injection is followed by flushing with normal saline. In a typical sequence, a preset protocol is used where the mechanical index is lowered when the contrast starts to fill the right side to allow enough time for optimal visualization without rapid bubbles destruction.

1.7.1   Safety Profile, Indications, and Contraindications (Table 1.2)

Mild and transient side effects such as headache, parestesias, back pain, or mild allergic reactions are occasionally described but serious adverse events are very rare (0.01%), so the overall safety profile is excellent. However, following reports of a few deaths cases after contrast studies in patients with severe, acute cardiopulmonary conditions, the European Medicines Agency (EMEA) in 2004 introduced limitations for the use of SonoVue

TABLE 1.2. Contrast echocardiography: general indications and contraindications.

Indications:
- Improve LV function assessment if
  - ≥2 segments not well visualized
- Improve definition of LV structures
  - LV thrombus
  - Pseudoaneurysm
  - Apical or noncompaction CMP
  - LV tumor
- Enhance Doppler signal of aortic stenosis

Contraindications:
- Known intracardiac shunts
- Previous allergic reaction to the agent
- Ongoing or recent acute or unstable cardiac conditions*
  - Unstable angina/acute coronary syndrome
  - Acute or severe cardiac failure
  - Complex ventricular arrhythmia or at risk for QT prolongation arrhythmia
- Suspected or likely pulmonary vascular disease*
  - Severe emphysema
  - Pulmonary embolism
  - ARDS

CMP cardiomyopathy
*see text below

in Europe and the Food and Drugs Administration (FDA) in 2007 required a boxed warning for the use of perfluoropropane agents (Luminity, Optisone) in the United States. Also the patients were to be monitored during the study and for 30 min thereafter. To which extent these major events were related to the use of contrast agents is debatable since they occurred in unstable and high-risk patients. These contraindications have been removed by the FDA in 2008, though the warning of possible severe reactions and the need for 30 minutes monitoring in high risk patients are maintained.

1.8   CONTROLS AND SETTINGS - PRACTICAL TIPS

- Decide on:
  - Transducer frequency
    - Low frequencies for overweight, big-chest, emphysematous patients
    - High frequencies for young, thin-chest individuals
  - Fundamental versus second harmonic imaging
    - Second harmonic imaging is preferred as a rule
- 2D Adjustments and settings
  - Depth of field
    - A good routine is to use more depth to get a general view and then, if necessary, reduce it to accommodate the area of interest.
  - TGC
    - Modern machines have built-in automatic TGC but also offer manual fine-tuning with a group of levers which control the differential amplification of the reflected ultrasound according to the tissue depth at which it originates. In a typical configuration, there is a gradual increase in amplification from near- to distal field.
  - Sector width and position
    - The narrower the scan sector is the better the image. Use a wide sector to get a general view and then narrow on your area of interest.
- Spectral Doppler adjustments and settings
  - Decide on:
    - PW to localize the site of flow acceleration
    - CW to display high velocities
  - Adjust baseline and scale to fit the displayed velocity (Fig. 1.4).

- ○ Consider using high-speed sweep velocities (100 cm/s) for better detailing of the waveform and lower velocities (25 cm/s) to assess phasic changes (i.e., mitral flow respiratory variations in tamponade)
- ○ If necessary, use color Doppler for optimal positioning of the PW sample volume or CW line, then turn color off to increase the frame rate.
- Color Doppler adjustments and settings
  - ○ Use a gain level that will give full color display without painting areas devoid of flow (extracardiac, nonflow regions)
  - ○ Use a scale (Nyquist limit) in the range of 50–60 cm/s for routine qualitative color imaging (Fig. 1.5)
  - ○ Use the B/W suppress function to eliminate 2D imaging out of the color sector
  - ○ Narrow the sector to your area of interest.
- General:
  - ○ Have a good ECG tracing for cardiac cycle events timing and for digital capture.
  - ○ Liberally use varying depths of field, sector widths, and zooming to improve image quality and anatomical detail. 2D visualization should be done first followed by color and spectral Doppler imaging if appropriate.
  - ○ For TEEs and studies in emergencies, tape and/or acquire everything: you may not have the chance to repeat the study.

1.9 ARTIFACTS

Artifacts can represent a diagnostic challenge even for the experienced echocardiographer. It is not unusual for TEE or magnetic resonance imaging (MRI) studies to be requested because of artifactual echo findings.

The most frequently encountered artifacts are as follows:

- Near-field noise artifacts (Fig. 1.9)
  - ○ These are seen as a clutter of echoes in the LV apex. Occasionally, they are misdiagnosed as apical masses.
- Reverberation artifacts (Figs. 1.10–1.11)
  - ° Are related to strong reflectors such as prosthetic valves, ribs, or pericardium. Generally, they appear as either linear echoes, which are occasionally confused with a pathological structure such as an intimal flap, or a foreign body, or as multiple echoes extending from the target structure into the far field. Occasionally, the reflected ultrasound is bounced back and forth between the transducer and the

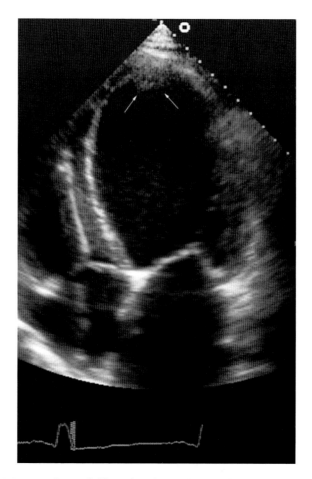

FIG. 1.9. Typical near-field artifact (*arrows*) mimicking a small protruding thrombus in apical 4-chamber view. In this case, the diagnosis was even more problematic since severe left ventricle systolic dysfunction was present. However, the overall appearance and lack of mobility as compared with the heart motion and a slight change in a near-field time-gain-compensation (*TGCs*), proved this to be an artifact.

        target, creating "ghosting" images, where two identical
        structures coexist in the same view.
- Side lobes artifacts
    ○ Strong reflectors at the periphery of the ultrasound beam
      can be displayed as originating within the main beam, so
      an existing structure appears or generates echoes in an
      unusual location.

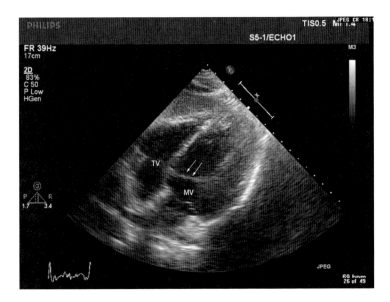

FIG. 1.10. Reverberation artifact, most probably due to a rib. A linear echogenic finding seems to be present in the LV cavity, below the MV in this subcostal view. Besides the unusual appearance, during real-time inspection of the acquired sequence, there was no relationship between this finding and the motion of the heart. *MV* mitral valve, *TV* tricuspid valve, *LV* left ventricle.

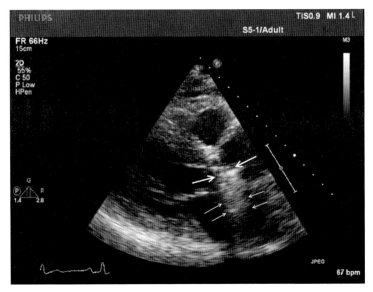

FIG. 1.11. Typical reverberations artifact appearing as multiple echoes (*thin arrows*) obscuring structures behind an aortic mechanical prosthetic valve (*thick arrows*).

1.9.1   Clues to Avoid and Recognize Artifacts

- Use lower power settings and harmonic rather than funda-
  mental imaging to reduce the odds of artifacts formation
- Think of an artifact whenever:
  - The image does not make sense
  - The overall appearance is unusual
  - The finding seems to be within the heart cavities or
    attached to a wall but does not move with the heart and
    has no motion of its own
  - It is at a distance from the transducer which is twice the
    one from the transducer to a highly echogenic structure
  - It is seen in one view only
- If an artifact rather than a true finding is suspected:
  - Lower the gains
  - Change the transducer frequency
  - Slightly change the transducer orientation
  - Look for a strong reflector that could explain artifact formation
  - Consult an experienced colleague

1.10   STANDARD VIEWS IN TRANSTHORACIC ECHOCARDIOGRAPHY

The standard views in transthoracic echocardiography are grouped
in parasternal, apical, subcostal, and suprasternal views according
to the position of the transducer. Ideally, the patient should be positioned in left lateral decubitus for the parasternal and apical views
and lying on his back for the subcostal and suprasternal views. In
unstable patients or during cardiopulmonary resuscitation (CPR),
only one or two views (subcostal and, if possible, apical) should be
attempted to immediately rule out critical pathologies, otherwise
all views should be attempted.

Transoesophageal views are discussed in Sect. 2.2.

1.10.1   Parasternal Views (Figs. 1.12–1.18)

Parasternal views are obtained with the transducer located immediately to the left of the sternum, generally in intercostal spaces 3–5
depending on body habitus. The imaging plane, as specified by the
marker on the transducer is aligned with the long axis of the ventricle for the parasternal long-axis (PSLA) view and then rotated at 90°
and tilted from the base toward the apex to obtain the parasternal
short-axis (PSSA) views of the heart. By convention, the heart is
displayed oriented with the apex toward the left side of the screen.

1.10.2   Apical Views (Figs. 1.18–1.21)

Apical views are obtained by positioning the transducer at the
apex, which can be either "looked for" in the fifth intercostal
space or located by palpation. The heart is displayed with the

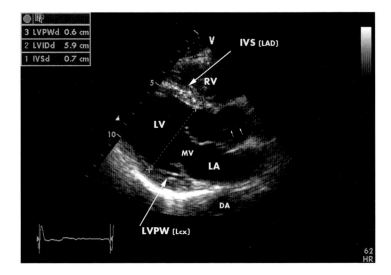

Fɪɢ. 1.12. End-diastolic frame in parasternal long-axis view, with identification of main anatomical structures and of coronary perfusion territories. Two-dimensional measurements for LV thickness and dimensions are also displayed. The closed aortic valve is seen as a fine line in the aortic root (*small arrows*). Note the nonspecific finding of strong and apparently thick pericardial reflection beyond the posterior wall in this normal subject without any suspicion of pericardial pathology. *DA* descending aorta, *IVS* interventricular septum, *LA* left atrium, *LAD* left anterior descending coronary artery, *Lcx* left circumflex coronary artery, *LVPW* left ventricular posterior wall.

apex toward the upper field of the screen, though some institutions use a reversed, more "true-to-anatomical orientation" display. To avoid foreshortening, a good technique is to move the transducer downwards and leftwards until the apex is lost, and then bring it back, until the apex is identified again. Rotation of the transducer counterclockwise will display first the apical 2-chamber and then the apical long-axis view.

1.10.3 Subcostal View (Fig. 1.22)

For this view, the transducer is positioned beneath the xyphoid appendix. Having the patient bend his knees to relax the abdominal wall and take a deep breath to flatten the diaphragm and lower the heart will improve the image. This view is of special importance in critically ill patient, since it may be the only available transthoracic view. In emergencies, it can rapidly confirm or rule out pericardial effusion or severe right ventricle (RV) enlargement suggestive of massive pulmonary embolism. It also allows

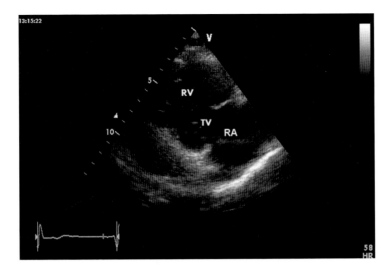

FIG. 1.13. Diastolic frame in PSLA view modified for the right ventricle inflow tract. The view is obtained starting from the standard PSLA view (Fig. 1.12) and tilting the transducer opposite to the left shoulder. May be the best available view for the tricuspid valve (*anterior and posterior leaflets*) and tricuspid regurgitant jet. *RA* right atrium, *TV* tricuspid valve, *PSLA* parasternal long axis.

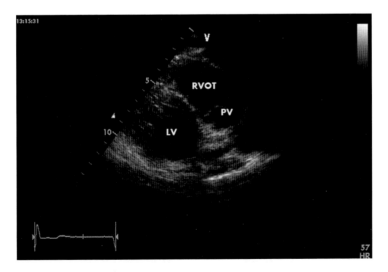

FIG. 1.14. Diastolic frame in PSLA view modified for the pulmonic valve and the main pulmonary artery. The view is obtained starting from the standard PSLA view (Fig. 1.12) and tilting the transducer toward the left shoulder. This view is not mandatory but it may complement the PSSA, basal-level view (Fig. 1.15). *PV* pulmonic valve, *RVOT* right ventricular outflow tract, *PSSA* parasternal short axis.

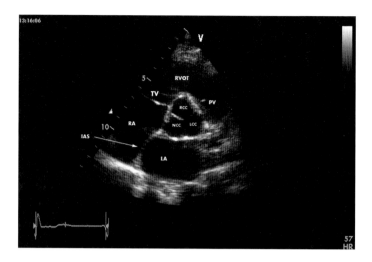

FIG. 1.15. Diastolic frame in **PSSA** view, basal level. The view allows simultaneous inspection of the aortic, pulmonic and tricuspid valve, interatrial septum, right ventricular outflow tract, and main pulmonary artery. *LCC* left coronary cusp, *NCC* noncoronary cusp, *RCC* right coronary cusp, *IAS* interatrial septum, *PSSA* parasternal short axis.

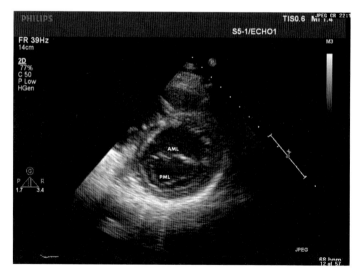

FIG. 1.16. Diastolic frame in PSSA at MV level showing the mitral leaflets in open position. The anterolateral and posteromedial commissures are positioned at 3 o'clock and 9 o'clock, respectively. *AML* anterior mitral leaflet, *PML* posterior mitral leaflet, *PSSA* parasternal short axis, *MV* mitral valve.

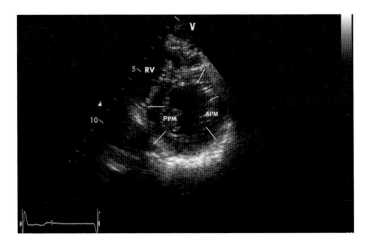

FIG. 1.17. End-systolic frame in **PSSA** view at papillary muscles level. The *white lines* mark the approximate boundaries between LV wall segments and their coronary supply, starting clockwise from a 9 o'clock position. *IVS (LAD)* left ventricular anterior wall (LAD), left ventricular lateral wall (Lcx), LVPW (PDA), left ventricular inferior wall (PDA), *APM* anterolateral papillary muscle, *PDA* posterior de-scending coronary artery, *PPM* postero-medial papillary muscle, *PSSA* parasternal short-axis.

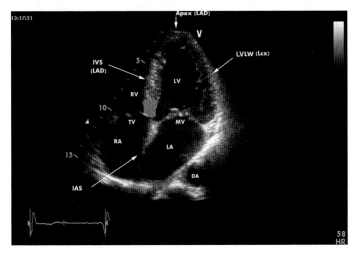

FIG. 1.18. End-systolic frame in apical 4-chamber view. The LV walls are identified with the corresponding coronary supply. The hachured area marks the basal inferior IVS which is vascularised by the right coronary artery. Note the very thin midportion of the interatrial septum (*fossa ovalis area*), which occasionally can be mistaken as a septal defect. *LVLW* left ventricular lateral wall, *IVS* interventricular septum.

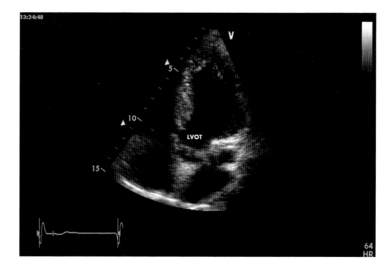

FIG. 1.19. End-diastolic frame in apical 5-chamber view. This view is obtained from the apical 4-chamber view position by tilting the transducer anteriorly. The outflow tract area is thus opened, allowing cardiac output measurements by combined two-dimensional and pulse wave Doppler imaging (see Appendix A). *LVOT* left ventricular outflow tract.

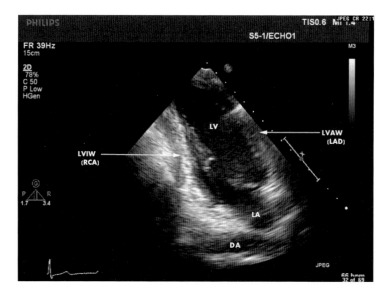

FIG. 1.20. End-diastolic frame in apical 2-chamber view. The LV walls are identified with the corresponding coronary supply. The descending aorta is occasionally visualized in long-axis in this view. *LVAW* left ventricular anterior wall, *LVIW* left ventricular inferior wall.

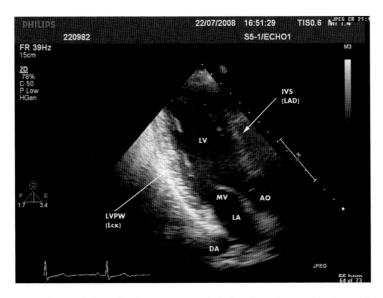

FIG. 1.21. End-diastolic frame in apical 3-chamber (*long-axis*) view. *AO* ascending aorta.

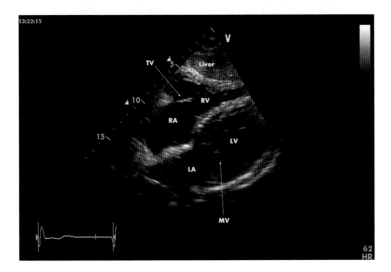

FIG. 1.22. Mid-diastolic frame in subcostal view. Chambers size and contractility and any significant pericardial effusion can all be quickly assessed in this view.

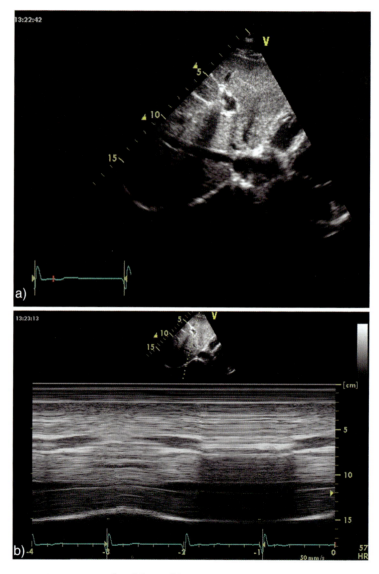

Fig. 1.23. IVC visualized by mild counterclockwise rotation and right-wards tilting of the transducer from the subcostal position. The diameter and the respiratory variations are assessed at about 1 cm from the junction with the right atrium. **a** two-dimensional image. **b** M-mode imaging demonstrating complete IVC collapse during inspiration, characteristic for low right atrial pressures. *IVC* inferior vena cava.

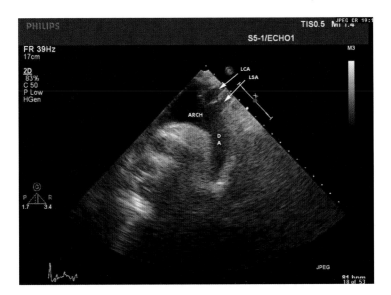

FIG. 1.24. Suprasternal view. The arch, left-side neck vessels, and the proximal descending aorta are clearly demonstrated. This view is not a routine one in emergency echocardiography unless aortic dissection is suspected. *LCA* left carotid artery, *LSA* left subclavian artery.

visualization of the inferior vena cava and, thus, assessment of right heart pressures (Fig. 1.23).

1.10.4 Suprasternal View (Fig. 1.24)

This is not a mandatory routine view but should be attempted whenever aortic enlargement or dissection is suspected. The patient should lie on his back with some neck hyperextension to allow proper transducer positioning.

References

1. de Jong N. Mechanical index. *Eur. J. Echocardiogr.* 2002;3(1):73–74.
2. Lang, RM, Mor-Avi V, Zoghbi WA, Senior R, Klein AL, Pearlman AS. The role of contrast enhancement in echocardiographic assessment of left ventricular function. *Am. J. Cardiol.* 2002;90(10A):28J–34J.
3. Stewart MJ.Contrast echocardiography. *Heart* 2003;89(3):342–348.

Chapter 2
Emergency Echocardiography

This chapter provides an overall view of the increasing contribution of echocardiography in the management of acutely ill patients and of its impact on outcome. Emphasis is put on the role of echocardiography in typical critical care situations and a diagnostic algorithm is suggested for immediate echocardiographic triage and monitoring of unstable patients. Techniques such as transesophageal and hand-held echocardiography are discussed in detail and a step-by-step practical guide of transesophageal imaging is provided, supported by relevant figures from real-life studies.

2.1 GENERAL OUTLOOK

2.1.1 Modalities

Echocardiographic studies in critically ill patients are generally performed bedside or in the acute assessment bay either as:

- Transthoracic study using:
  - Mainframe machine
  - Portable unit
  - Hand-held unit
- Transesophageal study using:
  - Mainframe machine
  - Portable unit

The information to be derived and the "logic of the study" are similar irrespective of the technique used. Specific indications, limitations and technical issues for transesophageal and hand-held echocardiography are detailed below.

A. Chenzbraun, *Emergency Echocardiography*, DOI: 10.1007/978-1-84882-336-5_2,

2.1.2 Clinical Scenarios and Indications for Use of Echocardio-graphy in Critically Ill Patients

An urgent echocardiographic study in an unstable patient may be required in the following clinical scenarios:

1. *Hemodynamic instability and/or hypoxemia of unclear aetiology*.
    (a) As a general rule, a hemodynamically unstable patient should be promptly assessed with echocardiography since this may provide an immediate understanding of the case. Mainly, a targeted echo assessment will allow the assignment of the patient to a broad pathophysiological category, which will guide subsequent management. This information is frequently more useful and comprehensive than the data obtained with invasive measurements, which often offer little on the mechanism of patient's deterioration. A general workflow approach for *Immediate Echocardiographic Triage* (IMET) is outlined in Fig. 2.1
    (b) Within this category there are two clinical situations which are recognized as indication for "emergency echocardiography."[1]
        (i) Suspected tamponade
        (ii) Pulseless electrical activity (PEA) can be the presenting symptom for:

    • Tamponade
    • Massive pulmonary embolism
    • Acute massive internal hemorrhage (e.g., ruptured aortic aneurysm)
    • Tension pneumothorax

2. *Critically ill patients due to non-cardiac illness* where, however, cardiac function and left ventricular (LV) filling status assessment may be crucial to guide fluid resuscitation, for example:
    (a) septic shock and
    (b) diabetic ketoacidosis.

3. *Relatively stable patients* with known or suspected acute cardiac pathology where echocardiography is necessary for further management and risk stratification.

The degree of "urgency" for an echocardiographic assessment in these cases may vary from emergency to scheduled pre-discharge evaluation. Typical examples in this category include:

1. Stable patients after successful resuscitation
2. Selected cases of acute coronary and chest pain syndromes
3. Aortic dissection

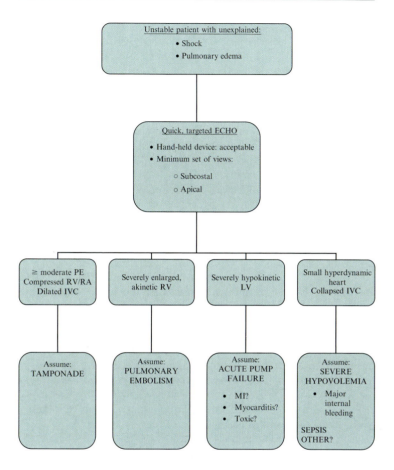

FIG. 2.1. Immediate Echocardiographic Triage (*IMET*) algorithm. Diagnostic criteria for specific scenarios including use of echocardiography during resuscitation are discussed further in the text.

4. Massive pulmonary embolism
5. Infective endocarditis
6. Acute native valves pathology
7. Prosthetic valves malfunction
8. Acute embolic events

A review of various studies on the use of echocardiography in critically ill patients[2–5] shows a quite consistent pattern, with the main conditions to benefit from an echo-guided approach listed below:

- Hemodynamic instability
- Sepsis
- Source of emboli
- Suspected aortic dissection
- Various

There is a wide consensus on the impact of the echo studies on the further management of these patients with most authors reporting an extremely positive input which translates in a change in therapy in 30–60% of cases even in patients who had invasive hemodynamic monitoring.

Although the clinical picture can be complex and different pathologies can coexist in a given patient, from a practical standpoint, rather standard scenarios can be expected (Table 2.1). Close review of the listed situations reveals that most of them have specific and occasionally divergent therapeutic approaches which would be very difficult to decide upon without echocardiographic information.

"Pre-echo" clinical knowledge of the case is essential in order to know what to look for and what to do with the echocardiographic results. The importance of familiarizing oneself with the case and understanding it before placing the transducer on the patient's chest cannot be overemphasized. The final diagnosis has to integrate all data using sound clinical judgment. Finally, a decision based on an echocardiographic evaluation *should be taken only if the study quality is deemed satisfactory for diagnostic purposes and the person performing it is trained and competent enough in using echocardiography.*[1] Flawed information may be more damaging than lack of information altogether.

While an emergency bedside study should aim to be as complete as possible, it is expected to be less detailed, of lesser quality and to include fewer measurements than a routine elective one due to a variety of factors:

- Limited echocardiographic windows
- Inability to position the patient for optimal imaging
- Bright room lighting
- Need to perform a short, "targeted" study due to patient instability or discomfort
- Use of a portable echocardiographic machine of less quality than a big unit
- Limited echocardiographic experience of the operator

However, the information listed below is essential and *should be actively sought by operator.*

TABLE 2.1. Typical scenarios requiring urgent echocardiographic assessment in critically ill patients.

Clinical scenario	Diagnostic question	Management question
Hypotension/shock	Hypovolemia? Pump failure? Inappropriate vasodilatation?	Fluid challenge? Vasoconstrictors/inotropes? CVP/Swan–Ganz monitoring?
Severe dyspnea	Cardiac versus noncardiac etiology • LV function – Systolic *and* diastolic • Valvular heart disease • Pericardial disease	Cardiac or noncardiac case?
Severe cardiomegaly	Cardiac cavities enlargement? Pericardial fluid?	
Systemic embolism	Intracardiac source of emboli	Anticoagulation?
Suspected pulmonary embolism	RV enlargement/failure Thrombus visualization (by TEE)	Thrombolysis Embolectomy
Deterioration in a patient with a prosthetic valve	Stuck valve Endocarditis Regurgitation	
Suspected tamponade	Hemodynamic impact of pericardial fluid	Need for pericardiocenthesis

(continued)

TABLE 2.1. (continued)

Clinical scenario	Diagnostic question	Management question
Suspected aortic dissection	Confirm Dg	Conservative versus emergent surgical approach
	Assess:	Need for AVR
	• involvement of ascending aorta	
	• pericardial/mediastinal fluid	
	• aortic regurgitation	
Hemodynamic deterioration in AMI	LV/RV function	Diuretics/inotropes/vasodilators
	Mechanical AMI complications	
	• MR	IABP
	• AVSR	Emergency surgery
	• Free wall rupture	
	• Dynamic LVOT obstruction	
Resuscitated sudden cardiac death	LV function	
	Pericardial fluid	
	Pulmonary embolism	
	Aortic dissection	

AMI acute myocardial infarction, *AVR* aortic valve replacement, *AVSR* acute ventricular septal rupture, *CVP* central venous pressure, *MR* mitral regurgitation, *LVOT* left ventricular outflow tract, *IABP* intraortic balloom pump, *RV* right ventricular, *LV* left ventricular, *TEE* transesophageal echocardiography

- LV
  - Size
  - Contractility
    - Global
    - Regional
  - Filling pattern
    - Suggestive of underfilled ventricle
    - Suggestive of high filling pressures
- Right ventricular (RV)
  - Size
  - Contractility
- Pericardial fluid
  - Amount
  - Evidence for tamponade
- Significant valvular pathology
- Pulmonary hypertension
- Any major pathological finding

A typical study should begin with an attempt at trans-thoracic imaging. It is the responsibility of the operator to decide whether the information obtained is satisfactory or more advanced techniques such as contrast or transesophageal echocardiography are needed.

2.2 TRANSESOPHAGEAL ECHOCARDIOGRAPHY IN THE CRITICALLY ILL PATIENT

Transesophageal echocardiography rapidly entered into clinical use starting with the 1980s. Its specific diagnostic advantages as compared with transthoracic echocardiography (TTE) (see below) derive from the positioning of the transducer into the esophagus, in the proximity of the heart (Fig. 2.2), thus allowing unimpeded imaging from a posterior-to-anterior view and the use of high frequencies providing better resolution.

2.2.1 TEE Imaging Advantages

- Interrogation of posterior cardiac structures generally not well imaged with TTE:
  - Pulmonary veins
  - Atrial appendages
  - Descending aorta
- Better imaging of difficult and/or small targets such as:
  - Vegetations
  - Prosthetic valves

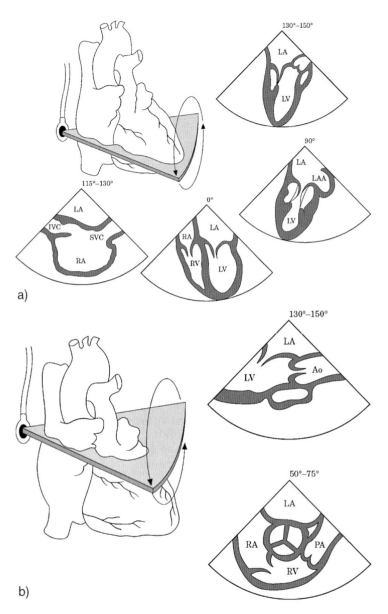

FIG. 2.2. Imaging planes and typical views of cardiac structures at standard esophageal positions and transducer angles. Although the transducer is situated posterior to the heart, the image is displayed as seeing the cross-sectional view from an anterior position. Left-sided structures are displayed on the right side of the screen and posterior structures are displayed in the upper part. **a** Mid-low esophageal positions, **b** mid-high esophageal

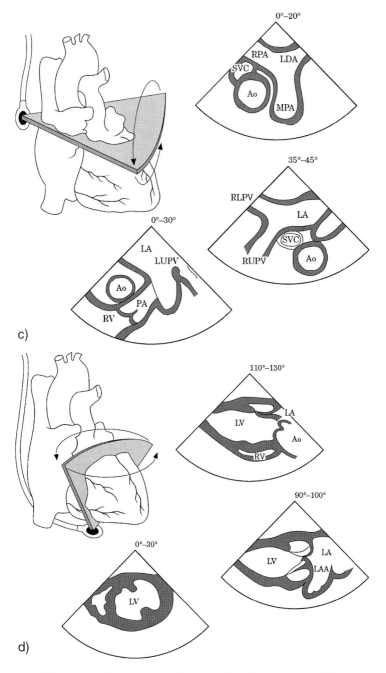

FIG. 2.2. (continued) positions, **c** high esophageal positions, and **d** transgastric positions. Adapted with permission from Flachskampf et al.[7]

2.2.2 TEE "First Line" Indications Are Summarized Below and Are Detailed in Available Guidelines[6,7]

- Aortic pathology
  - Acute aortic syndromes
  - Aortic trauma
- Infective endocarditis (selected cases)
  - Positive diagnostic
  - Complications
- Prosthetic valves assessment
  - Obstruction
  - Regurgitation
  - Prosthetic valve endocarditis
- Suspected high-risk pulmonary embolism
- Source of systemic/cerebral emboli
  - Intracardiac masses/clots
  - Intracardiac shunts
  - Aortic atheromas
- Valvular pathology
  - Equivocal TTE studies
  - Pre-repair assessment
- Imaging guiding during procedures
  - Atrial septal defect (ASD)/patent foramen ovale (PFO) closure
  - Mitral valve balloon valvuloplasty
  - Percutaneous aortic valve replacement
- Hemodynamic monitoring during surgery
- Poor quality TTE imaging when the echocardiographic information is considered essential for management.

2.2.3 TEE Versus TTE in the Critically Ill Patient

The tendency exists to consider transesophageal echocardiography (TEE) as the first step for echocardiographic imaging in intensive care units (ICU) patients. Indeed, due to limitating factors in these patients, TTE imaging failure rates of up to 40% have been previously quoted.[8] However, following the continuous improvement in image quality with modern systems and the use of harmonic imaging, TTE can actually provide useful information in a surprisingly high percentage of patients with a failure rate possibly as low as 10–15%.[9] Moreover, some areas such as LV apex or the aortic valve in the presence of a prosthetic mitral valve are usually better visualized by transthoracic echocardiography. Cavities size and ventricular contractility are also occasionally more accurate by TTE. Accordingly, it is our policy to always attempt a transthoracic study first and to continue with a TEE, if:

- Image quality is unsatisfactory for a confident diagnosis or
- The clinical question in itself is a "TEE-first line" indication (see above).

2.2.4 TEE Contraindications, Safety and Precautions

In critically ill patients, TEE has a special role due to its input in some of the encountered pathologies and to the higher likelihood of limited quality transthoracic studies in this population. A large body of literature has documented the excellent yield and safety profile of TEE in intensive care patients.[2,10–13] Except for some esophageal pathologies and cervical spine instability, there are no absolute contraindications for TEE. Hemodynamic instability and acute conditions as such *are not a contraindication*, in fact, if appropriate, they may be an indication for TEE diagnostic work-up. The TEE technique in critically ill patients is similar to the one used in stable, elective ones, however, some precautions are to be taken:

- In hemodynamically unstable or hypoxemic patients, it may be preferable to have the sedation performed, or at least supervised, by an anesthetist. The "threshold"for requiring this assistance depends on the operator's expertise and the severity of the case.
- In mechanically ventilated patients, achieving the appropriate level of sedation is generally the responsibility of the ICU team. Removing the naso-gastric tube before the procedure is recommended to facilitate probe advance and improve imaging. Also care should be exercised not to dislodge the endotracheal tube during intubation of the esophagus and when withdrawing the probe.
- As a rule, a TEE in an unstable patient should be performed by an experienced practitioner and not by a beginner or an occasional operator.

2.2.5 TEE Examination Protocol

- Individual routines vary but the concept of following a study protocol is crucial in order to avoid missing important information. Guidelines on how to perform TEE and how to assess specific pathologies exist[7,14] and may be adapted to personal preferences.
- If no recent TTE study is available, the TEE should be complemented, if possible, by even a quick TTE scan.
- Though *a complete and systematic study should be attempted in all cases*, it is a good routine in patients who are unstable or tolerate the procedure poorly, to start with the "target" (i.e., prosthetic valve, aorta, LV function) and then continue with a full study so that if the procedure has to be prematurely terminated, the important information has been acquired.

• The examination can be either "view guided," that is, the operator follows an orderly sequence of standard views as in a transthoracic study, or "structure guided" where each structure is fully interrogated in appropriate views, before the next structure is targeted. It is our opinion that a "view guided" approach is generally superior since it is less likely to omit certain views and miss important information, while a "structure guided" approach may be more appropriate in unstable patients.

A suggested sequence for a TEE "view guided" examination protocol is detailed below. Recommended probe positions and transducer angles are orientative and have to be adapted to the patient's specific anatomical particularities. A standard view of a given structure is "expected" but not certain to be found at a certain angle and depth, so scanning has to be performed in a true "windscreen wiper" manner until the required view is achieved. As a general rule, try first to understand the two-dimensional anatomy and then use color Doppler.

Position I: Mid-esophageal at 0° (Fig. 2.3).

This is a good starting view to give an overall "feel of the heart" and detect pericardial effusion or extracardiac compressing masses.

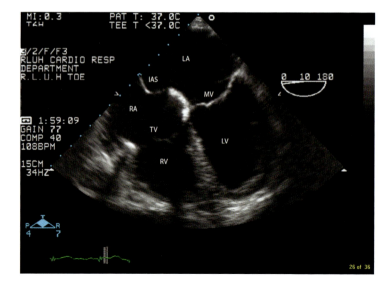

FIG. 2.3. Systolic frame of an apical 4-chamber view obtained from a mid-esophageal position with the transducer at 0°.

– Equivalent transthoracic view: apical 4-chamber view
– Structures: atria, ventricles, mitral and tricuspid valves (TV)
– Suggested manoeuvres at this level are:

• Retroversion of the probe tip using the big wheel may help to avoid a short-axis cut with vertical hearts in this view.
• Rotation of the probe shaft counter-clockwise and clockwise to scan the left atrium (LA) leftwards and rightwards, respectively, and the mitral valve (MV) from the septal to the lateral aspect of the annulus.
• Clockwise rotation with slight advancement of the probe may optimize the TV and the IAS as well.

Position II: High esophageal at 0° (Fig. 2.4).

There are three levels here to be structure targeted through gradual withdrawing of the probe.

– Aortic valve level (roughly equivalent to a 5-chamber view) for left ventricular outflow tract (LVOT) and anterior segments of the MV
– Left atrial appendage (LAA) and left upper pulmonary vein (LUPV) level
– Superior vena cava (SVC), ascending aorta and main pulmonary artery (MPA) level

Position III (Fig. 2.5): Back to mid-esophageal level, slightly advancing the probe to "lose" the aortic valve with counter-clockwise rotation to bring the MV in the centre of the image. Scan from 40° to 90° for MV interrogation.

– Equivalent transthoracic views: apical 2-chamber view
– Structures: MV, LV, LA, LAA
– Once at 90°, clockwise rotation will open the right ventricular outflow tract (RVOT) and the MPA.

Position IV (Fig. 2.6): Back to mid- to high-esophageal position until the aortic valve (AV) becomes visible again. There are three transducer angulations to be used here:

◦ 0°
▫ Equivalent transthoracic view: basal parasternal short-axis view
▫ Structures: TV, AV, RVOT, PV, left main coronary artery, LAA
◦ 120°
▫ Equivalent transthoracic view: parasternal long-axis view

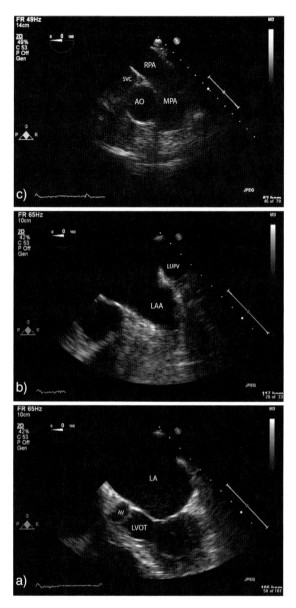

FIG. 2.4. Transesophageal echocardiography (*TEE*) imaging at 0° with gradual withdrawing of the probe from mid- to high- (**a–c**) esophageal positions. **a** Aortic valve level position for left ventricular outflow tract (*LVOT*) and anterior mitral valve (*MV*) segments. **b** Left atrial appendage position. The left upper pulmonary vein is visualized on its left (right on screen), separated by a ridge. **c** Proximal ascending aorta position with good imaging of the proximal aortic root and the superior vena cava in cross-sectional view and the main pulmonary artery in long-axis view.

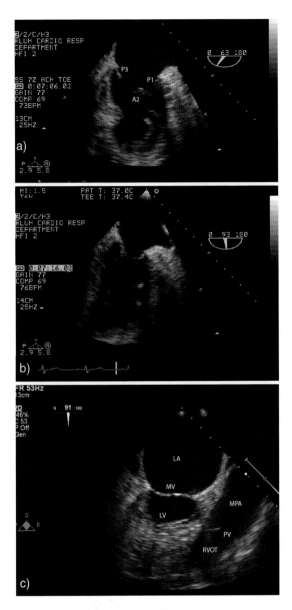

FIG. 2.5. Transesophageal echocardiography (*TEE*) scanning from 40° to 90° at mitral valve level. **a** Bicommissural view to identify the mitral valve segments. The anterior leaflet central segment is seen between the posterior mitral leaflet posterior and anterior segments in this early-diastolic frame. **b** 2-Chamber view demonstrating the anterior and inferior left ventricular (*LV*) walls. **c** Rightwards (*clockwise*) rotation from position **b** brings in the right ventricular outflow tract, pulmonic valve, and proximal main pulmonary artery.

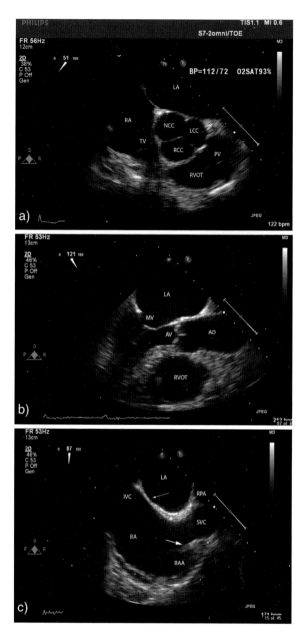

Fig. 2.6. Transesophageal echocardiography (*TEE*) scanning starting at aortic valve level in short-axis view and continuing to a bicaval view. **a** 20°–40°: short-axis view of the aortic valve, allowing clear identification of the cusps. The tricuspid and the pulmonic valves, the left atrial appendage and, occasionally, the proximal left coronary system are also seen at this

  □ Structures: MV, proximal interventricular septum (IVS), aortic root and AV
○ 90° with clockwise rotation (bicaval view)
  □ Structures: SVC, interior vena cava (IVC), right atrial appendage (RAA)

Position V: Transgastric (Fig. 2.7).
○ At 0°
  □ Equivalent transthoracic view: PSSA
  □ Structures: LV and RV
○ At 90°–120°
  □ Equivalent transthoracic views: parasternal long-axis (PSLA) and 2-chamber view
  □ Structures: LV, MV, subvalvular apparatus

Position VI (Fig. 2.8): Withdraw to a mid-esophageal level and then rotate shaft posteriorly in a counter-clockwise direction with transducer at 0° until the thoracic descending aorta is visualized in a short-axis cut. Advance the probe until the aorta is lost at diaphragmatic level and then withdraw slowly until it changes course and disappears again at distal arch level. Shaft rotation may be necessary to follow a tortuous aorta. When pathology is noted, the level should be recorded using the

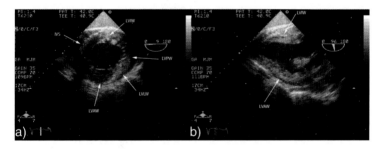

FIG. 2.7. Transgastric views. These are essential if the main query is left ventricle contractility or mitral subvalvular pathology, but are not mandatory if this information is available from the transthoracic study. **a** Cross-sectional view allowing good visualization of ventricular walls at mid-ventricle level. **b** Long-axis view.

FIG. 2.6. (continued) level. **b** 120°: long-axis view of the left ventricular outflow tract, mitral and aortic valve and aortic root. **c** 90° with rightwards rotation of the transducer. The junctions of the two vennae cavae and the interatrial septum at fossa ovalis level (*thin arrow*) are visualized at this level. *Thick arrow*: crista terminalis.

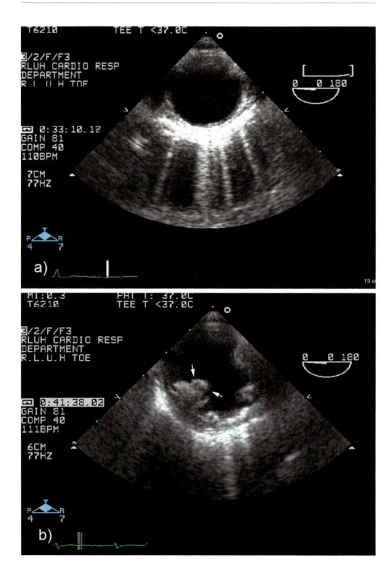

Fig. 2.8. Cross-sectional view of the descending thoracic aorta. This view is mandatory for type B aortic dissection, intramural hematoma or aortic atherosclerosis. **a** Normal aorta. **b** Severe atherosclerosis of descending aorta with complex plaque and mobile atheroma (*arrows*), found as an incidental finding in a patient undergoing TEE before cardioversion; this underscores the importance of routine scanning of the aorta.

TABLE 2.2. Frequently encountered clinical scenario and recommended structure-targeted modular approach in unstable patients when a brief TEE examination is required.

Dg. module	"Not to be missed" echo targets	Essential views
(a) Hemodynamic instability	• LV/RV contractility • LV/RV dimensions • LV Doppler filling pattern by PW Doppler of mitral inflow	I, IV, VI
(b) Difficulty to wean from ventilator	• LV/RV contractility • MR presence • R L shunt (PFO)	I, IV, VI
(c) Aortic dissection	• Aortic root • Descending aorta	II, III, VII
(d) Massive pulmonary embolism	• RV size and function • Pulmonary artery size and scanning for clot • TR	I, II, IV

PFO patent foramen ovale, *TR* tricuspid regurgitation, *RV* right ventricle, *LV* left ventricle, *MR* mitral regurgitation, *PW* pulsed wave

distance markers on the probe shaft. Long-axis cuts should also be used for detailed imaging of wall pathology.

If the patient is unstable use a diagnostic module approach (Table 2.2) and start with a "structure targeted" study to address the main clinical question. Complete the study if possible, after obtaining the critical information.

2.3   HAND-HELD ECHOCARDIOGRAPHY IN THE CRITICALLY ILL PATIENT

Hand-held echocardiography, formally referred to as hand-carried ultrasound (HCU), is an ultrasound diagnostic modality whose role and indications are under continuous review reflecting evolving technological advances. A 2002 report of the American Society of Echocardiography emphasizes HCU as an extension of physical examination while acknowledging that revisions of this document may be required to reflect ongoing technologically driven developments. A wealth of data has accumulated to support the reliability of HCU echocardiography when compared with standard platform systems with best results for two-dimensional information and somewhat less for color Doppler.[15]

2.3.1   What Is a HCU?

A HCU system will typically fulfil the following criteria:

- Light (usually < 6 lbs)
- Easily portable, without the need of a carrying trolley
- Battery powered
- Significantly cheaper than a conventional system

2.3.2   Particularities of HCU Imaging

Because of the basic capabilities of first generation devices and the initial scope of HCU use mainly as a convenient aid to bedside examination, some study limitations are accepted as compared with a standard examination:

- Study duration:
  - brief (<5–10 min)
- Scope:
  - targeted to confirm or rule out a major finding or clinical diagnosis:
    - Pericardial effusion
    - Severe systolic dysfunction
    - Severe hypertrophy
    - Severe valvular pathology
- Imaging modalities:
  - possibly limited (i.e., spectral Doppler may not be available)
- Image quality:
  - possibly limited:
    - small screen size
    - restricted color capabilities
- Report:
  - not standardized, limited, findings may be only briefly mentioned in the patient's notes
- Images storage:
  - optional, thus without the possibility of later review
- Accepted minimal training level of the operator: Level 1

However, with continuous technological advances, some of these limitations may become irrelevant and the capabilities of new models tend to blur the differences between a high-end HCU and a portable conventional system (Figs. 2.9 and 2.10).

2.3.3   HCU Echocardiography in the Critically Ill

HCU devices should be used in critically ill patients mainly for screening purposes and assessment at the time of the first evaluation. Because of their portability and good two-dimensional images, they may be the preferred tool for an instant, emergency assessment as outlined in Fig. 2.1. The results of the scan may

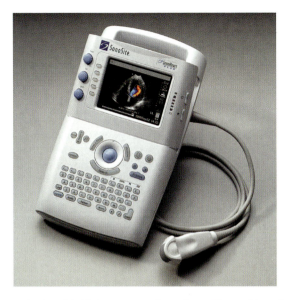

FIG. 2.9. Light, hand-held SonoHeart Elite echocardiographic unit.

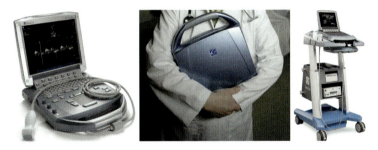

FIG. 2.10. Newer generation M-Turbo unit, still light and portable but suitable for trolley-mounting and carrying as well. (Images used in Figs. 2.9 and 2.10 are courtesy of SonoSite, Inc., 21919 30th Drive SE, Bothell, WA 98021-3904).

immediately point to the underlying pathology, for example, empty ventricles, tamponade or severe systolic dysfunction, making a comprehensive standard examination not necessary at that moment though it may still be required at a later stage. Despite the expected quality limitations in difficult to image ICU patients, HCU scanning was found to have a diagnostic accuracy and therapeutic impact similar to those of conventional systems, mainly for two-dimensional imaging.[16,17]

2.4 CONTRAST ECHOCARDIOGRAPHY IN THE CRITICALLY ILL PATIENT

Contrast echocardiography can be performed either as a "conventional study" with agitated saline, for right heart visualization, or using transpulmonary agents for left heart imaging.

2.4.1 "Conventional" Contrast Echocardiography for Right-to-Left Shunts

Right-to-left shunts occur mainly at interatrial septal level through a PFO or previously unrecognized ASD and, occasionally, at pulmonary level through arteriovenous fistulae, either isolated or in association with liver disease (hepatopulmonary syndrome). A PFO is present in about 25–30% of the general population; the magnitude and occurrence of the shunt may increase with pulmonary hypertension, which is frequently encountered in ICU patients due to either cardiac or primary lung conditions. A right-to-left shunt should be suspected in cases of persistent hypoxemia (see Sect. 2.4) or unexplained embolic stroke. Color Doppler is not sensitive enough, especially for transthoracic studies and small shunts, and a formal contrast study should be performed when a right-to left shunt is suspected. Rapid injection of agitated saline through an antecubital or central vein is the most practical way to check whether a right-to-left shunt is present. The solution is prepared by vigorous mixing of 10 ml normal saline with a small amount (~0.5 ml) of air using two syringes, preferably of Luer lock type, connected by a three-way stopcock. Apical 4-chamber imaging by either TTE (Fig. 2.11) or TEE is the view of choice, though a bicaval view should be used as well with TEE. A first injection is generally performed without provocation and, in cooperative patients, is repeated with provocation using:

- A Valsalva manoeuvre with the patient instructed to build the pressure during injection and to abruptly release it when the contrast reaches the right heart
- A forceful cough at the time of right heart opacification

The efficacy of a provocation manoeuvre during TEE can be checked by visualizing a brief bowing of the IAS towards the LA due to the transient raise of the right atrium (RA) pressures. Some patients are not able to perform an effective Valsalva manoeuvre or to cough during a TEE study. A high-quality TTE with good provocation should, therefore, complete a negative TEE or even may obviate the need for it if presence or absence of the shunt was the only query.[18] In ventilated patients, manual inflation of the lungs, followed by

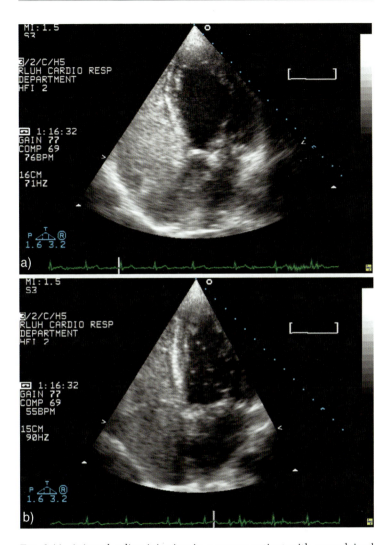

FIG. 2.11. Agitated saline injection in a young patient with unexplained transient ischemic attack (*TIA*). **a** Good contrast injection without provocative maneuver fully opacifies the right heart without any passage of bubbles to the left heart. **b** Repeat injection with a vigorous cough shows a moderate amount of bubbles in the left cavities, making this a positive test for right-to-left shunt.

abrupt release, may be equivalent to a Valsalva manoeuvre.[15] If left cavities opacification does occur, both its timing and magnitude should be noted. A shunt is diagnosed if 1 bubble is seen in the left heart, though some studies required 3 bubbles for clinical significance.[19] The appearance of contrast later than five cycles after right heart opacification suggests intrapulmonary rather than intracardiac shunt. The number of bubbles observed in the left heart defines the shunt magnitude with some authors considering 10 and others 30 bubbles as the cut-off for a large shunt.[19] Of note, the magnitude of the shunt as defined by the number of bubbles transiting to the left heart is a functional assessment different from the anatomical size of the PFO, which generally is assessed with TEE or during surgery.

Other uses for right-sided contrast echocardiography

Agitated saline injection has been also shown to enhance the Doppler signal of tricuspid regurgitation (TR). This technique may be used to improve the accuracy of pulmonary artery pressure measurement in patients with mild or poorly defined TR signal.

2.4.2 Contrast Echocardiography for Left Ventricular Opacification

The technical aspects, indications and contraindications of contrast studies using transpulmonary agents for better visualization of the LV have been discussed in Sect. 1.6. As mentioned, poor LV imaging may be an even more relevant factor in critically ill patients. Ventricular cavity opacification using contrast echocardiography has been shown to dramatically improve left ventricular function assessment by transthoracic studies in the intensive care unit setting[20-23] and thus may obviate the need for a TEE.

Reference

1. Stewart WJ, Douglas PS, Sagar K, et al. Echocardiography in emergency medicine: a policy statement by the American Society of Echocardiography and the American College of Cardiology. The Task Force on Echocardiography in Emergency Medicine of the American Society of Echocardiography and the Echocardiography TPEC Committees of the American College of Cardiology. *J Am Soc Echocardiogr.* 1999;12(1):82–84.
2. Chenzbraun A, Pinto FJ, Schnittger I Transesophageal echocardiography in the intensive care unit: impact on diagnosis and decision-making. *Clin Cardiol.* 1994;17(8):438–444.

3. Denault AY, Couture P, McKenty S, et al. Perioperative use of transesophageal echocardiography by anesthesiologists: impact in noncardiac surgery and in the intensive care unit. *Can J Anaesth.* 2002;49(3):287–293.

4. Bruch C, Comber M, Schmermund A, et al. Diagnostic usefulness and impact on management of transesophageal echocardiography in surgical intensive care units. *Am J Cardiol.* 2003;91(4):510–513.

5. Stanko LK, Jacobsohn E, Tam JW, De Wet CJ, Avidan M. Transthoracic echocardiography: impact on diagnosis and management in tertiary care intensive care units. *Anaesth Intensive Care.* 2005;33(4):492–496.

6. Douglas PS, Hendel RC, Patel RM, et al. ACCF/ASE/ACEP/ASNC/ SCAI/SCCT/SCMR 2007 appropriateness criteria for transthoracic and transesophageal echocardiography: a report of the American College of Cardiology Foundation Quality Strategic Directions Committee Appropriateness Criteria Working Group, American Society of Echocardiography, American College of Emergency Physicians, American Society of Nuclear Cardiology, Society for Cardiovascular Angiography and Interventions, Society of Cardiovascular Computed Tomography, and the Society for Cardiovascular Magnetic Resonance endorsed by the American College of Chest Physicians and the Society of Critical Care Medicine. *J Am Coll Cardiol.* 2007;50(2):187–204.

7. Flachskampf FA, Decoodt P, Fraser AG, Daniel WG, Roelandt JR Guidelines from the Working Group. Recommendations for performing transesophageal echocardiography. *Eur J Echocardiogr.* 2001;2(1):8–21.

8. Cook CH, Praba AC, Beery PR, Martin LC. Transthoracic echocardiography is not cost-effective in critically ill surgical patients. *J Trauma.* 2002;52(2):280–284.

9. Beaulieu Y, Marik PE. Bedside ultrasonography in the ICU: part 1. *Chest.* 2005;128(2):881–895.

10. Slama MA, Novara A, Van de Putte P, et al. Diagnostic and therapeutic implications of transesophageal echocardiography in medical ICU patients with unexplained shock, hypoxemia, or suspected endocarditis. *Intensive Care Med.* 1996;22(9):916–922.

11. Vieillard-Baron A, Slama M, Cholley B, Janvier G, Vignon P. Echocardiography in the intensive care unit: from evolution to revolution? *Intensive Care Med.* 2008;34(2):243–249.

12. Vignon P, Mentec H, Terré S, Gastinne H, Guéret P, Lemaire F. Diagnostic accuracy and therapeutic impact of transthoracic and transesophageal echocardiography in mechanically ventilated patients in the ICU. *Chest.* 1994;106(6):1829–1834.

13. Hwang JJ, Shyu KG, Chen JJ, et al. Usefulness of transesophageal echocardiography in the treatment of critically ill patients. *Chest.* 1993;104(3):861–866.

14. Shanewise JS, Cheung AT, Aronson S, et al. ASE/SCA guidelines for performing a comprehensive intraoperative multiplane transesophageal echocardiography examination: recommendations of the American Society of Echocard-iography Council for Intraoperative Echocardiography and the Society of Cardiovascular Anesthesiologists Task Force for

Certification in Perioperative Transesophageal Echocardiography. *J Am Soc Echocardiogr.* 1999;12(10):884–900.

15. Beaulieu Y, Marik PE. Bedside ultrasonography in the ICU: part 2. *Chest.* 2005;128(3):1766–1781.

16. Goodkin GM, Spevack DM, Tunick PA, Kronzon, I. How useful is hand-carried bedside echocardiography in critically ill patients? *J Am Coll Cardiol.* 2001;37(8):2019–2022.

17. Vignon P, Chastagner C, Françoiset B, et al. Diagnostic ability of hand-held echocardiography in ventilated critically ill patients. *Crit Care.* 2003;7(5):R84–R91.

18. Clarke NR, Timperley J, Kelion AD, Banning AP. Transthoracic echocardiography using second harmonic imaging with Valsalva manoeuvre for the detection of right to left shunts. *Eur J Echocardiogr.* 2004;5(3):176–181.

19. Pinto FJ. When and how to diagnose patent foramen ovale. *Heart.* 2005;91(4):438–440.

20. Makaryus AN, Zubrow ME, Gillam LDet al. Contrast echocardiography improves the diagnostic yield of transthoracic studies performed in the intensive care setting by novice sonographers. *J Am Soc Echocardiogr.* 2005;18(5):475–480.

21. Nash PJ, Kassimatis KC, Borowski AG, et al. Salvage of nondiagnostic transthoracic echocardiograms on patients in intensive care units with intravenous ultrasound contrast. *Am J Cardiol.* 2004;94(3):409–411.

22. Yong Y, Wu D, Fernandes V, et al. Diagnostic accuracy and cost-effectiveness of contrast echocardiography on evaluation of cardiac function in technically very difficult patients in the intensive care unit. *Am J Cardiol.* 2002;89(6):711–718.

23. Reilly JP, Tunick PA, Timmermans RJ, Stein B, Rosenzweig BP, Kronzon I. Contrast echocardiography clarifies uninterpretable wall motion in intensive care unit patients. *J Am Coll Cardiol.* 2000;35(2):485–490.

Chapter 3
Echocardiography
in the Hypotensive Patient

Hypotension is a frequent scenario in unstable patients. The differential diagnosis between systolic ventricular failure and inadequate filling of the left ventricle can be challenging. This chapter offers a practical integrated echocardiographic diagnostic approach, which makes invasive assessment unnecessary in most cases. Other entities which can include hypotension as part of their clinical presentation are discussed as well. Section 3.5 is dedicated to management of cardiac tamponade, including both echocardiographic diagnosis and guiding of pericadiocenthesis.

3.1 INTRODUCTION

Persistent hypotension is defined as systolic blood pressure (BP) <90 mmHg and may reflect a shock syndrome. The following clinical features emphasize the hemodynamic impact of low BP and underline the urgency of diagnosis and treatment especially in cases with borderline-low BP values:

- Known baseline high BP values
- Sudden/rapidly evolving BP fall
- Mean BP <60 mmHg
- Clinical evidence of systemic vasoconstriction/hypoperfusion
  - Cold/clammy/cyanotic extremities
  - Restlessness, confusion
  - Declining urinary output
  - Metabolic acidosis
- Occurrence during an acute coronary syndrome
- Accompanying pulmonary congestion

A. Chenzbraun, *Emergency Echocardiography*, DOI: 10.1007/978-1-84882-336-5_3,
© Springer-Verlag London Limited 2009

Occasionally, the reason for hypotension is obvious: dehydration, bleeding, anaphylaxis, vasodilators overuse, and extreme bradycardia. Otherwise, understanding why the patient is actually hypotensive is crucial and should be addressed as soon as possible. This is where echocardiography is irreplaceable as a first-line diagnostic technique and should be able to pinpoint the mechanism of hypotension to be one of the following:

- Left ventricle (LV) systolic dysfunction
- LV underfilling
  - Hypovolemia
  - Right ventricle (RV) dysfunction
- Acute valvular pathology
- Tamponade

3.2 LV SYSTOLIC DYSFUNCTION AS A CAUSE OF HYPOTENSION

Chronic LV dysfunction even severe does not generally translate into acute clinical hypotension; if severe LV hypocontractility is seen in an unstable hypotensive patient, the LV impairment has to be assumed to be acute, or a precipitating/worsening factor has to be sought:

- Acute coronary syndrome
- Intravascular hypovolemia with relative ventricular underfilling
- Uncontrolled arrhythmia
- Acute nonischemic myocardial depression
  - Acute myocarditis
  - Recent prolonged CPR
  - Severe hypoxaemia and/or acidosis
  - Drug induced
    - Ca- or β-blockers overdose

From an echocardiographic point of view, the diagnosis of systolic dysfunction is generally a qualitative one where the degree of impairment is graded as mild, moderate, or severe based on a subjective assessment of ventricular hypokinesis. The visual assessment of ventricular hypocontractility can be supplemented by looking for additional findings as detailed below. Quantitative assessment as calculation of ejection fraction or cardiac index is not generally necessary for immediate management but can be obtained (Appendix B).

Practical tips to remember:

- Mild degrees of LV systolic dysfunction can be missed or masked by use of inotropes and vasodilators, but LV hypocontractility severe

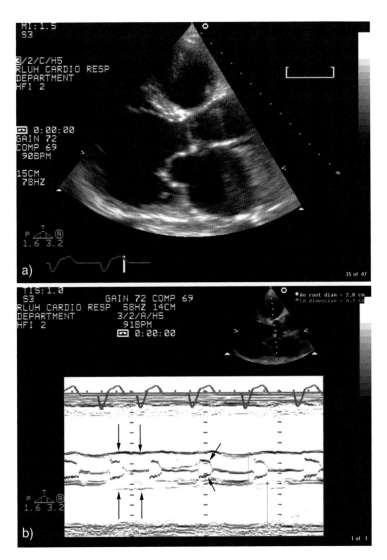

FIG. 3.1. M-mode supportive findings of severely decreased left ventricle (*LV*) contractility in a patient with dilated cardiomyopathy **a** two-dimensional imaging of the in parasternal long-axis view, showing a dilated, globular, and severely hypokinetic LV **b** M-mode scan at aortic root level. Note the flat motion (*long arrows*) of the aortic root secondary to the decreased stroke volume and the premature beginning of closure of the aortic valve leaflets (*short arrows*) reflecting the inability of the ventricle to maintain an effective flow rate throughout the ejection period.

enough to cause hypotension or low cardiac output should be easily recognized.

- The actual degree of LV systolic impairment can be misinterpreted with:
  - Poor quality images without endocardial visualization,
  - Rapid/irregular heart rhythm,
  - Wide LBBB,
  - Ventricular paced rhythm.
- Segmental wall motion abnormalities suggest ischemic etiology, while diffuse hypokinesis is associated with cardiomyopathy or advanced valvular disease, but:
  - Diffuse hypokinesis can be present in coronary artery disease patients with triple vessel disease and diffuse ischemic damage.
  - Acute myocarditis can present with regional wall motion abnormalities.
- If in doubt, look for additional echocardiographic signs of severe LV systolic dysfunction:
  - Reduced motion amplitude of the aortic wall,
  - Early closure pattern of the aortic valve (Fig. 3.1),
  - Decreased mitral annulus systolic motion:
    - Amplitude <12 mm by M-mode and
    - Velocity <8 cm/s by tissue Doppler.[1]
- If you do not feel comfortable with images' quality, suggest:
  - TEE with emphasis on transgastric views (esophageal views may be misleading due to oblique cuts) and
  - Contrast echocardiography for LVO.
- Many instances of acute severe systolic dysfunction are *at least partially reversible*. This is true both for acute coronary syndromes after the initial stunning (especially if the patient undergoes revascularization) and for nonischemic etiologies. In fact, *improvement of the systolic dysfunction after the acute event is frequent enough to warrant a repeat echocardiographic assessment at a later stage*. Taking major therapeutic decisions such as suitability for aggressive therapy or need for a defibrillator or biventricular pacemaker, based on the LV contractility, assessed only once during the acute phase may be misleading.

3.3 LV UNDERFILLING AS A CAUSE OF HYPOTENSION

3.3.1 Background

Hypotension due to obvious hypovolemia such as bleeding, vomiting, or diarrhea is usually a self-evident diagnosis, which does not require echocardiographic assessment especially in patients without a cardiac background.

A more complex situation arises when hypotension or low cardiac output occur in the setting of LV systolic dysfunction. This may reflect a combination of both pump failure and inadequate LV filling. The diseased ventricle is highly dependent on optimal end-diastolic filling to maintain systolic performance. Various acute conditions may be complicated by relative hypovolemia due to diuretics use and fluid restriction. *Assessing the volemic status of hypotensive patients with LV dysfunction is one of the most frequent challenges in clinical practice*. Moreover, patients with hypertension, diabetes, recent myocardial infarction, or sepsis have stiff LVs which require higher than normal end-diastolic filling pressures. *In particular, for acute myocardial infarction, it has been shown using invasive measurements that a relatively high pulmonary capillary wedged pressure (PCWP) of ≈ 15–20 mmHg may be necessary for an adequate cardiac output*[2] *and similar recommendations exist for septic patients*.[3] The differential diagnosis between critical hypotension due to severe pump failure only or secondary to a combination of systolic dysfunction and relative LV underfilling is of vital importance since the latter may benefit from cautious fluid challenging. Classically, the determination of the filling status relied on invasive right heart pressures monitoring using a balloon-tipped flow-directed Swan-Ganz catheter and assuming that the measured pulmonary capillary wedged pressure reflects the left atrial pressure. However, the use of Swan-Ganz catheters requires a degree of expertise not always available and is fraught by specific potential complications. Moreover, the left-sided pressures as measured with a Swan-Ganz catheter may have a limited correlation only with the filling status since they reflect not only the absolute volume status but chamber compliance as well. In practice, we witness a continuous decline in the use of invasive hemodynamic monitoring in these patients and increasing reliance on echocardiographic assessment instead.[4]

3.3.2 Echocardiographic Assessment of Hypovolemia and Filling Status

The echocardiographic assessment of volemia and filling status comprises two elements (see also Appendix C):

3.3.2.1 *Evaluation of Effective Central Blood Volume*

This is the amount of blood present in the thoracic vessels and available for ventricular filling. The normal central blood volume

(CBV) represents ≈ 10% of the total blood volume[4] and it can be reduced either by absolute loss or by abnormal redistribution (Table 3.1). The net result of a significantly decreased CBV is a fall in ventricular preload and a possible reduction of cardiac output. The echocardiographic hallmarks of a low CBV (marked cyclic respiratory variations of the venae cavae) and underfilled LV (Fig. 3.2) are summarized in Table 3.2.

3.3.2.2   Evaluation of LV Filling Status

The LV filling depends on both the CBV and the ventricular stiffness. As detailed above, a diseased, noncompliant ventricle can be relatively underfilled even with a normal CBV. This paragraph deals with the echocardiographic assessment of the ventricular filling status using flow- and tissue Doppler.

For flow-Doppler evaluation, the mitral valve diastolic flow pattern is obtained in apical 4-chamber view with the pulsed wave sample placed at mitral leaflets tips level. The resulting velocity

TABLE 3.1. Main etiologies of central blood volume (CBV) reduction.

Absolute loss
• bleeding
• dehydration
• vomiting, diarrhea

Intravascular redistribution
• sepsis
• anaphylaxis
• increased intrathoracic pressures

Third space redistribution
• Massive edema, ascites, anasarca

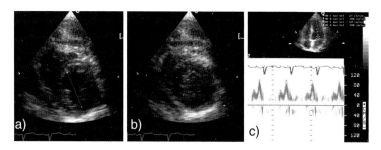

FIG. 3.2. Two-dimensional and Doppler findings in a patient with severe hypotension and oliguria due to hypovolemia. (**a**) Small (3.7 cm) end-diastolic diameter, (**b**) end-systolic cavity obliteration, and (**c**) *E/A* ratio markedly <1 (see text below).

TABLE 3.2. Main echocardiographic findings in hypovolemic patients.

Small, hyperdynamic heart
E/A < 1 pattern
Small (<20 mm) IVC with >50% respiratory diameter variations
Increased (>60%) respiratory variations in the diameter of SVC moni tored by TEE in mechanically ventilated patients[4]

[a]Can be obscured by tachycardia and fusion of *E* and *A* waves

waveform has an early peak (E) at the time of the early filling phase and an end-diastolic one (A) following the atrial contraction (Fig. 1.4). The velocities reflect the instantaneous atrioventricular gradient at any given time; the areas (time-velocities integrals) of the E and A components reflect the relative volumetric filling in early and late diastole. *In young healthy individuals, the peak velocity and velocity-time integral are bigger for the E component reflecting vigorous relaxation and physiological early-diastolic filling preponderance.* With age, the E/A peak velocities ratio reverses leading to an E/A ratio <1 which reflects impaired relaxation and a greater contribution of the atrial contraction to overall ventricular filling; within certain limits, this is an age-dependent physiological process. A similar reversal occurs with acute or chronic myocardial damage such as ischemic heart disease, cardiomyopathy, or hypertrophic states since active relaxation is impaired in all these cases even before systolic impairment occurs. However, *for atrial contribution to become predominant, atrial contraction has to be mechanically effective, that is, the patient has to be in sinus rhythm and the end-diastolic filling pressures have to be relatively low. An apparently normal E/A >1 ratio in a patient with LV systolic dysfunction or organic heart disease is unexpected and suggests increased late-diastolic pressures with subsequent failure of the atrial contribution to filling* (Fig. 3.3). This "pseudonormalization" of the E/A ratio has long been described to occur at a range of LVEDP values ≥15 mmHg.[5] The deceleration time will be also decreased in these cases, reflective of a rapid cessation of early filling due to abrupt rise in the intraventricular pressures. In a more extreme variant, the E wave will be high and brisk with a markedly reduced deceleration time (<140 ms) and a diminutive A wave: this is known as a restrictive pattern and suggests very high filling pressures. A distinction has to be made between the chronic restrictive pattern in patients with restrictive cardiomyopathy and the possibly transient restrictive pattern (restrictive physiology) in patients with systolic dysfunction and fluid overload. The discussion in this chapter refers mainly to acute assessment of the filling status in unstable patients. For a summary of echocardiographic assessment of diastolic function, see Appendix C.

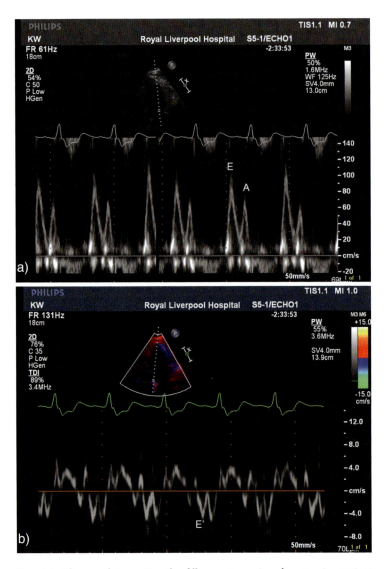

FIG. 3.3. Flow- and tissue-Doppler filling patterns in a hypotensive patient with severely decreased left ventricle (*LV*) systolic contractility. The *E/A* ratio = 1.6. The patient is unlikely to benefit from fluid challenge. In this clinical context, TDI is not routinely necessary to confirm raised filling pressures, unless the use of *E/A* ratio is not practical (*see* Limitations in text). In this case, the *E/E'* ratio was 25, confirming elevated diastolic pressures. **a** Pulsed wave flow-Doppler with the sample volume at the tips of the mitral valve. **b** Tissue-Doppler with the sample volume at the septal side of the mitral annulus.

- *In practical terms, faced with a clinically hypotensive patient:*
  - If E/A < 1 (Fig. 3.2c), assume relative hypovolemia even in the presence of systolic dysfunction.
  - If E/A > 1(Fig. 3.3), hypovolemia is less likely.
- *Limitations: this straightforward assessment is not usable with:*
  - *Rapid or slow heart rates*
  - *Mitral valve disease*
  - *Nonsinus rhythm*
  - *Recent atrial fibrillation*: It may be a limitation even when the patient is in sinus rhythm since it can be followed by periods of atrial stunning which will result in small A velocities irrespective of the filling pressures.

These limitations may be partially circumvented by the use of tissue Doppler[6] as explained in Sect. 1.5. A high-velocity E wave on the mitral valve Doppler flow velocity signal should be matched in normal individuals by a vigorous E′ wave on the tissue Doppler signal at mitral annulus level since both reflect forceful relaxation. With pseudonormalization due to increased diastolic pressures, the E wave velocity increases to reflect the high instantaneous LA to LV gradient after mitral valve opening but the actual LV expansion will be less forceful and E′ wave velocity actually decreases (Fig. 3.3).

An E/E′ ratio more than 15 in this context is definitely indicative of high filling pressures while a ratio of 8–15 is less specific and E/E′ less than 8 does not support the diagnosis.

Either the lateral or the medial aspect of the mitral annulus can be used, though using the medial aspect may increase sensitivity.

A simple step-by-step approach to assess the filling status in hypotensive patients is outlined in Fig. 3.4.

The Doppler patterns provide *a snapshot of the hemodynamic status of the patient at the time of the study*. A restrictive looking pattern may change to a low pressures one after good diuresis, so repeat Doppler studies offer a simple, noninvasive way to monitor changes in patients filling status (Fig. 3.5).

3.4 RV DYSFUNCTION AS A CAUSE OF HYPOTENSION

Severe RV failure can induce hypotension or low cardiac output due to underfilling of the LV.

The clinical picture will be of right heart failure and hypotension and the echocardiographic picture will include an enlarged, hypokinetic RV, and possibly a hyperdynamic LV.

RV contractility is more difficult to assess than LV contractility but severe cases should be recognized, especially since they are

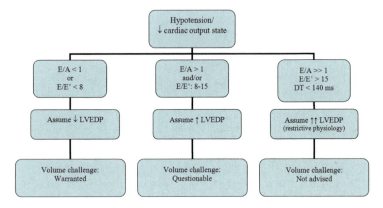

FIG. 3.4. Quick algorithm to assess filling status and the need for volume challenge using mitral valve flow- and tissue-Doppler patterns. The *E/E'* ratio is necessary when *E/A* ratio cannot be used or in borderline cases.

associated with RV enlargement as well (Fig. 3.6). Also, as for the LV, a reduced tricuspid annulus velocity (<8 cm/s) supports the diagnosis of RV dysfunction.[7] An important issue is to differentiate between an RV failing because of primary acute RV pathology (e.g., acute inferior + RV myocardial infarction) and an RV failing because of an acute rise in pulmonary artery pressure, that is, acute cor pulmonale such as pulmonary embolism. Besides the overall clinical picture, the following echocardiographic data can help in the differential diagnosis (Table 3.3).

3.5 TAMPONADE AS A CAUSE OF HYPOTENSION

Rapid accumulation of even a moderate amount of pericardial fluid or slow accumulation of a large amount can bring about a situation of restricted ventricular filling with high filling pressures and decreased cardiac output. This represents cardiac tamponade which, when full-blown, will present as hypotension with pulsus paradoxus, possibly syncope, dyspnea, tachycardia, and clinical evidence of peripheral hypoperfusion including decreased urinary output and metabolic acidosis.

3.5.1 Echocardiographic Diagnostic of Tamponade

This diagnostic implies:

• Demonstration of pericardial fluid
• Demonstration of tamponade physiology

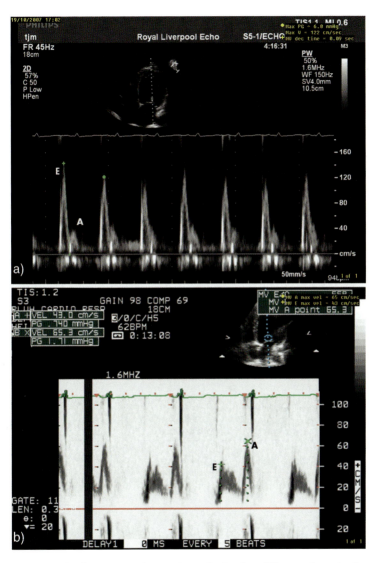

FIG. 3.5. Pulsed wave Doppler tracings obtained at different times in the same patient with severe left ventricle (*LV*) dysfunction. **a** On admission, with the patient in decompensated cardiac failure. Note the high and brisk *E* wave and the diminutive *A* wave, indicative of a restrictive pattern with markedly elevated filling pressures. **b** After vigorous diuresis and clinical improvement, the *E/A* ratio is now less than 1, with an expanded *A* wave. The changes parallel the decrease in the LV filling pressures.

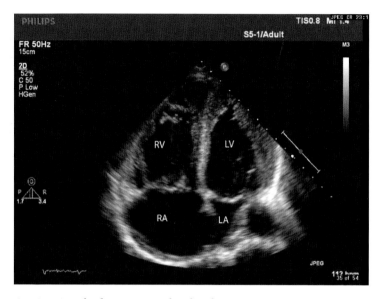

FIG. 3.6. Systolic frame in apical 4-chamber view in a patient with severe chronic cor pulmonale and chronic hypotension, worsened during an acute infectious episode. The right ventricles was severely dilated and hypokinetic, while the left ventricle was with normal size and function.

TABLE 3.3. Echocardiographic features to in primary and secondary acute RV failure

	Enlarged, hypokinetic RV	LV inferior akinesis	PHT[a]
Primary RV failure	Yes	Yes	No
(Acute) cor pulmonale	Yes	No	Yes

[a]It is generally accepted that severe pulmonary hypertension (*PHT*), that is, mean PAP ≥ 40 mmHg. is in general a chronic condition since even a previously intact right ventricle (*RV*) would not be able to acutely generate this degree of PHT and would fail

3.5.1.1 Demonstration of Pericardial Fluid

The presence of pericardial effusion is demonstrated as an echo-free (i.e., black) cavity surrounding the whole heart or overlying some areas only and limited by a bright parietal pericardial layer. In the absence of adhesions, a large pericardial effusion will tend to be circumferential while small effusions accumulate mainly posterior to the heart in the recumbent patient. Moderate and even large effusions may accumulate slowly without evidence of tamponade (Fig.

3.7). For a rough assessment, a pericardial space of up to 1 cm width represents a small effusion, a 1–2 cm width represents a moderate pericardial effusion, and >2 cm width represents a large effusion (Table 3.4).[8] The pericardium behind the left atrium is kept taut by the pulmonary veins so the left atrium is generally spared though the presence of fluid around it is possible and its appearance may be confusing (Fig. 3.8). A small pericardial space with some echogenicity may suggest either organized pericardial fluid or, if situated anteriorly, pericardial fat. The pericardial fluid is generally echo-free but fibrin filaments or clots can be present. Occasionally, a pericardial effusion has to be differentiated from a pleural one: The presence of the fluid posterior to the descending aorta in the parasternal long axis view supports the diagnosis of pleural effusion (Fig. 3.9).

3.5.1.2 Demonstration of Tamponade Physiology

The main echocardiographic signs of tamponade[9–13] are discussed and summarized below (Table 3.5).

Right Atrial Collapse

Due to its thin walls and low intracavitary pressures, the right atrium is the first cavity to be compressed with fluid accumulation in the pericardial sac. As such, right atrial collapse or inversion is a highly sensitive sign, picking up even minimal elevations in the intrapericardial pressure. However, since it has also been described in patients with small pericardial effusion and no hemodynamic confirmation of tamponade, its specificity for clinical use is low, especially as an isolated finding. The inversion of the atrial wall starts at ventricular end-diastole when the intra-atrial pressure is at its lowest during atrial relaxation. Persistence of atrial wall inversion during ventricular systole is considered to strengthen the diagnosis of tamponade since intrapericardial pressure tends to diminish at the time of ventricular contraction when cardiac dimensions decrease (Fig. 3.10a).

Diastolic Right Ventricular Collapse

Starting in the thinner-walled RV outflow tract area, diastolic RV collapse occurs with further elevation of intrapericardial pressures. Thus, it is a more specific sign than right atrial collapse, while having a good sensitivity and signaling a more advanced degree of hemodynamic compromise. The echocardiographic appearance is quite typical, with one area of the RV free wall having a delayed diastolic expansion as compared with the adjacent segments (Fig. 3.10b).

Respiratory Variations of Mitral and Tricuspid Diastolic Velocities

During inspiration, the right heart filling augments to accommodate the increased venous return, thus limiting the LV filling, whose

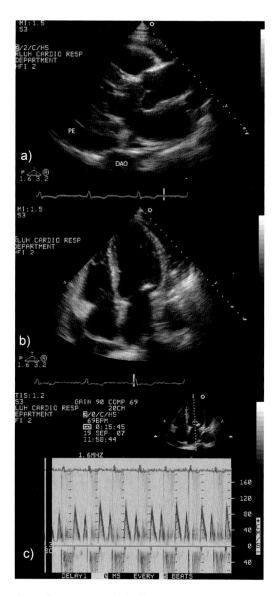

FIG. 3.7. Moderate-large pericardial effusion without echocardiographic evidence of tamponade. **a** Parasternal long-axis view early-diastolic frame demonstrating the typical extension of the fluid anterior to the descending aorta. Note the lack of right ventricular diastolic collapse. **b** Apical 4-chamber view end-diastolic frame showing the fluid mainly around the right atrium and the left ventricle (*LV*) lateral wall. Note the absence of right atrial inversion. **c** Pulsed wave Doppler recording of the mitral inflow showing minimal (<20%) respiratory variations in mitral flow velocity in this case of slowly accumulating effusion.

TABLE 3.4. Quantitative assessment of a pericardial effusion.

Pericardial space separation (cm)[a]	Expected effusion amount (ml)[b]
<1	300
1–2	500
>2	700

[a]Measurements are end-diastolic. Systolic separation only would indicate a nonsignificant pericardial effusion
[b]Orientative only and assuming circumferential distribution and normal-sized heart

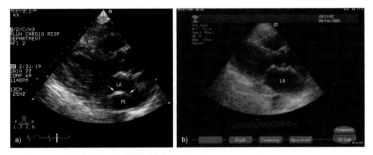

FIG. 3.8. Pericardial effusion causing left atrial tamponade in a patient with previous coronary artery bypass graft surgery. **a** A bright curved linear pericardial echo (*arrows*) delineates a localized pericardial effusion compressing the left atrium. Initially, it was thought to represent an intra-atrial structure. **b** Same patient after pericardial tap. The left atrium is now fully expanded without any posterior effusion.

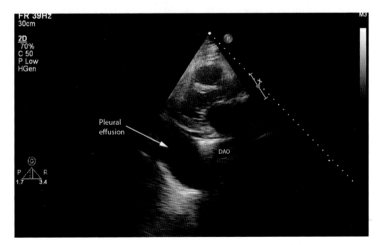

FIG. 3.9. Large left pleural effusion. Note the extension of the fluid posterior to the descending aorta. A small pericardial effusion is also present in this case, delineating the bright pericardium and extending anterior to the descending aorta.

TABLE 3.5. Accuracy of main echocardiographic findings in tamponade.

Echo cardiographic finding	Sensitivity (%)	Specificity (%)	Underlying physio-pathology
RA collapse	80–100	30–80	IP pressure ≥ RA pressure
RV collapse	70–80	90	IP pressure ≥ RV diastolic pressures
MV flow respiratory variations	77–90	80–88	Ventricular inter-dependence

IP intrapericardial pressure, *RA* right atrium, *RV* right ventricle, *MV* mitral valve

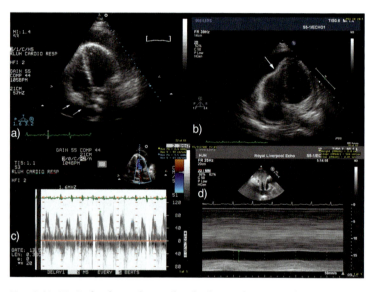

FIG. 3.10. Typical echocardiographic findings of tamponade in a patient with a large pericardial effusion. **a** Early-systolic frame in apical 4-chamber view. There is marked right atrium collapse (*arrows*) with almost total obliteration of the right atrium cavity. **b** Diastolic frame in apical 4-chamber view. There is typical appearance of localized compression (*arrow*) of the right ventricular free wall which fails to expand as compared with adjacent segments. **c** Pulsed wave Doppler recording at mitral valve level. There is 33% change from the tallest to the lowest E wave. **d** Subcostal view showing a dilated (3 cm) inferior vena cava without any change in diameter during respiration, indicative of elevated right atrium pressure. This "flat" pattern can be visually identified in the two-dimensional image and clearly checked on the M-mode scan.

concomitant expansion is impeded by the raised intrapericardial pressures; an opposite process occurs during expiration. These changes are reflected by spectral Doppler interrogation which shows an increase of pulmonary and tricuspid velocities during inspiration, with concomitant aortic and mitral velocities decrease and an opposite phenomenon during expiration. The degree of velocity change has been quantified mainly for the mitral and tricuspid flows. Since ventricular interdependence exists in normal individuals as well and some degree of respiratory changes may be physiologic, only changes of >20% are considered consistent with tamponade hemodynamics. This criterion is very popular but is not reliable with atrial fibrillation. Also, it is not specific for tamponade, being described with pleural effusion as well and in patients with chronic lung disease.

Inferior vena cava plethora with decreased respiratory variations indicates high right atrial pressures (Fig. 3.10d). As such this is not a finding specific for tamponade but its absence would make the diagnosis unlikely.

Caveats in the Clinical Diagnosis of Tamponade:

- Tamponade does not have to be a sudden, all-or-nothing catastrophic event, but frequently, it is rather a continuous clinical and hemodynamic spectrum ranging from mild hemodynamic impairment suggested by tachycardia and some oliguria to a full-blown shock picture.
- A normal BP reading can be misleading in a previously hypertensive patient.

Caveats in the Echocardiographic Diagnosis of Tamponade:

- Deceivingly small amounts of pericardial fluid can result in tamponade if rapidly accumulated. This is true especially for traumatic or iatrogenic tamponade.
- Not all the echocardiographic signs of tamponade (see above) have to be present for a valid diagnosis: right heart cavities collapse may be minimal in patients with raised right-sided pressures due to chronic lung disease or with stiff RV due to malignant infiltration (Fig. 3.11). Also, previous thoracic surgery with resulting adherences may promote a loculated and potentially misleading appearance of the effusion (Fig. 3.8).
- Tamponade features soon after cardiac surgery may be atypical. In these patients, a high suspicion index of tamponade in the presence of otherwise unexplained hemodynamic deterioration and of a demonstrable effusion, by either TTE or TEE, has been proven more valuable than the classical echocardiographic findings.[14,15]

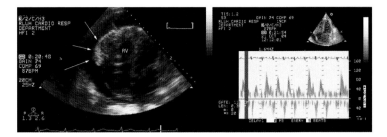

Fig. 3.11. Tamponade due to malignant pericardial effusion. There is no diastolic collapse of the right ventricular free wall which is covered and infiltrated by malignant tissue (*arrows*). The pulsed wave mitral valve Doppler shows marked respiratory variations consistent with tamponade physiology.

3.5.2 Echocardiographic Guided Pericardiocenthesis

Whether elective or emergent, pericardiocenthesis should be echocardiographic guided whenever possible. Two-dimensional imaging immediately before and during the procedure serves two purposes:

3.5.2.1 Deciding on the Most Appropriate Site of Puncture and on Optimal Needle Orientation

The most frequently used approach is subcostal, with the needle oriented in the general direction of the left shoulder. Imaging from the subxyphoid area with the transducer draped in a sterile cover will confirm the best direction for the largest pericardial space from this position, while at the same time avoiding a transhepatic tract. The distance from the skin to the pericardium and the orientation of the transducer should be mentally noted and the needle should be inserted as attempting to prolong the central axis of the transducer. A good technique is to position a finger parallel to the transducer and then use it to guide the needle. In a different approach, echo scanning is used to identify the area where the pericardial space is widest and closest to the chest wall and perform the tap at that site. Excellent results are reported with this method, the apical window being by far the most frequently used.[16]

3.5.2.2 Confirming That the Needle Is Indeed in the Pericardial Space

The aspiration of a clear yellow fluid from a large effusion should leave no doubt about the correct position of the needle. However, heavily hemorrhagic effusions may present a problem. Trying to visualize the wire is unrewarding in many cases. The simplest way to verify that we are in the right place is to inject a small amount of

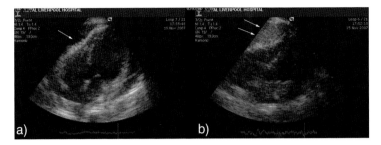

F<small>IG.</small> 3.12. Echo-guided pericardial tap. **a** Before injection, the pericardial effusion is seen as a black space (*arrow*) with right ventricular compression. **b** After injection of agitated saline, the pericardial space is filled with bright echoes (*arrows*) confirming the correct location of the needle.

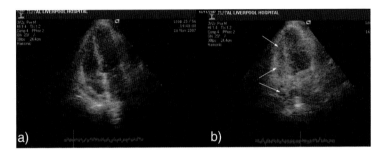

F<small>IG.</small> 3.13. Echo findings in a case of right atrial perforation during attempted pericardial tap. **a** Before injection, the cardiac cavities appear black, surrounded by a small amount of pericardial effusion. **b** After injection of agitated saline, there is immediate filling with bubbles of the right atrium and right ventricle (*arrows*), indicating right atrial perforation.

agitated saline, while an assistant images the effusion. The appearance of a cloud of small white echoes within the pericardial space will confirm intrapericardial position of the needle (Fig. 3.12), while opacification of the heart cavities will indicate intracardiac position (Fig. 3.13).

References

1. Elnoamany MF, Abdelhameed AK. Mitral annular motion as a surrogate for left ventricular function: correlation with brain natriuretic peptide levels. *Eur J Echocardiogr*. 2006;7(3):187–198.
2. Van de Werf F, Ardissino D, Betriu A, Cokkinos DV et al. Management of acute myocardial infarction in patients presenting with ST-segment

elevation. The Task Force on the Management of Acute Myocardial Infarction of the European Society of Cardiology. *Eur Heart J.* 2003;24(1):28–66.

3. Practice parameters for hemodynamic support of sepsis in adult patients in sepsis. Task Force of the American College of Critical Care Medicine, Society of Critical Care Medicine. *Crit Care Med.* 1999;27(3):639–660.

4. Vieillard-Baron A, Prin S, Chergui K, Dubourg O, Jardin F, et al. Hemodynamic instability in sepsis: bedside assessment by Doppler echocardiography. *Am J Respir Crit Care Med.* 2003;168(11):1270–1276.

5. Chenzbraun A, Keren A, Stern S. Doppler echocardiographic patterns of left ventricular filling in patients early after acute myocardial infarction. *Am J Cardiol.* 1992;70(7):711–714.

6. Ommen SR, Nishimura RA, Appleton CP, Miller FA, Oh JK, Redfield MM, Tajik AJ et al. Clinical utility of Doppler echocardiography and tissue Doppler imaging in the estimation of left ventricular filling pressures: a comparative simultaneous Doppler-catheterization study. *Circulation.* 2000;102(15):1788–1794.

7. Tuller D, Steiner M, Wahl A, Kabok M, Seiler C, et al. Systolic right ventricular function assessment by pulsed wave tissue Doppler imaging of the tricuspid annulus. *Swiss Med Wkly.* 2005;135(31–32):461–468.

8. Brockington GM, Schwartz TL, Pandian NG. Echocardiography in Pericardial Diseases. In: Marcus ML, Schelbert HR, Skorton DJ, Wolf GL (ed). Cardiac Imaging. 1991. W.B. Saunders Company, Philadelphia.

9. Appleton CP, Hatle LK, Popp RL. Cardiac tamponade and pericardial effusion: respiratory variation in transvalvular flow velocities studied by Doppler echocardiography. *J Am Coll Cardiol.* 1988;11(5):1020–1030.

10. Armstrong WF, Schilt BF, Helper DJ, Dillon JC, Feigenbaum H, et al. Diastolic collapse of the right ventricle with cardiac tamponade: an echocardiographic study. *Circulation.* 1982;65(7):1491–1496.

11. Gillam LD, Guyer DE, Gibson TC, King ME, Marshall JE, Weyman AE, et al. Hydrodynamic compression of the right atrium: a new echocardiographic sign of cardiac tamponade. *Circulation.* 1983;68(2):294–301.

12. Plotnick GD, Rubin DC, Feliciano Z, Ziskind AA, et al. Pulmonary hypertension decreases the predictive accuracy of echocardiographic clues for cardiac tamponade. *Chest.* 1995;107(4):919-924.

13. Materazzo C, Piotti P, Meazza R, Pellegrini MP, Viggiano V, Biasi S, et al. Respiratory changes in transvalvular flow velocities versus two-dimensional echocardiographic findings in the diagnosis of cardiac tamponade. *Ital Heart J.* 2003;4(3):186-192.

14. Faehnrich JA, Noone RB, Jr., White WD, et al. Effects of positive-pressure ventilation, pericardial effusion, and cardiac tamponade on respiratory variation in transmitral flow velocities. *J Cardiothorac Vasc Anesth.* 2003;17(1):45-50.

15. Price S, Prout J, Jaggar SI, Gibson DG, Pepper JR, et al. 'Tamponade' following cardiac surgery: terminology and echocardiography may both mislead. *Eur J Cardiothorac Surg.* 2004;26(6):1156-1160.

16. Tsang TS, Freeman WK, Barnes ME, Reeder GS, Packer DL, Seward JB, et al. Rescue echocardiographically guided pericardiocentesis for cardiac perforation complicating catheter-based procedures. The Mayo Clinic experience. *J Am Coll Cardiol.* 1998;32(5):1345-1350.

Chapter 4

Echocardiography in the Hypoxemic Patient

Unexplained hypoxemia can occasionally be related to right-to-left shunting through an unsuspected interatrial communication. This chapter deals with the role of echocardiography in persistently hypoxemic intensive care units (ICU) patients, without a clear cardiac or pulmonary etiology.

Isolated hypoxemia without accompanying heart failure or obvious cardiac pathology is unlikely to be cardiac in origin. However, *persistent hypoxemia in a patient with right ventricular infarction,*[1] *or mechanically ventilated,*[2] *should raise the suspicion of right-to-left shunt through a patent foramen ovale (PFO)* (Fig. 4.1). Using color Doppler or contrast, a PFO can be diagnosed with either a good quality TTE or, if needed, a TEE (see Sect. 6.4). Selected cases may benefit from a transcatheter closure as the only therapeutic measure.[3-5]

A. Chenzbraun, *Emergency Echocardiography,* DOI: 10.1007/978-1-84882-336-5_4,
© Springer-Verlag London Limited 2009

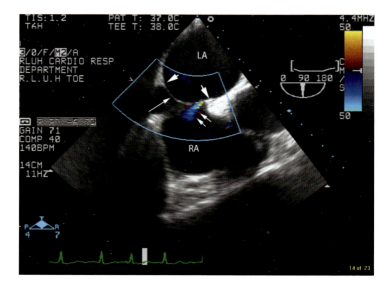

FIG. 4.1. Transesophageal echocardiography (*TEE*) demonstration of a patent foramen ovale (*PFO*) (*short arrows*) using color Doppler in this slightly modified bicaval view. The thin fossa ovalis area (*long thin arrow*) is clearly seen between the boundaries of septum secundum (*short arrows*).[6]

References

1. Silver MT, Lieberman EH, Thibault GE. Refractory hypoxemia in inferior myocardial infarction from right-to-left shunting through a patent foramen ovale: a case report and review of the literature. *Clin Cardiol.* 1994;17(11):627–630.
2. Cujec B, Polasek P, Mayers I, Johnson D. Positive end-expiratory pressure increases the right-to-left shunt in mechanically ventilated patients with patent foramen ovale. *Ann Intern Med.* 1993;119(9):887–894.
3. Cox D, Taylor J, Nanda NC. Refractory hypoxemia in right ventricular infarction from right-to-left shunting via a patent foramen ovale: efficacy of contrast transesophageal echocardiography. *Am J Med.* 1991;91(6):653–655.
4. Nguyen DQ, Das GS, Grubbs BC, Bolman RM III, Park SJ. Transcatheter closure of patent foramen ovale for hypoxemia during left ventricular assist device support. *J Heart Lung Transplant.* 1999;18(10):1021–1023.
5. Kuch B, Riehle M, von Scheidt W. Hypoxemia from right-to-left shunting through a patent foramen ovale in right ventricular infarction: treatment by revascularization, preload reduction, and, finally, interventional PFO closure. *Clin Res Cardiol.* 2006;95(12):680–684.
6. Chenzbraun A, Pinto FJ, Schnittger I. Biplane transesophageal echocardiography in the diagnosis of patent foramen ovale. *J Am Soc Echocardiogr.* 1993;6(4):417–421.

Chapter 5
Echocardiography in Valvular Emergencies

Valvular emergencies present clinically as either primary hemodynamic instability or as part of another acute condition. This chapter summarizes the echocardiographic diagnosis of both native and prosthetic valves acute pathologies. Emphasis is given to both common and specific echocardiographic features as they relate to the underlying mechanism. Special situations such as acute myocardial infarction-related mitral regurgitation or prosthetic valve pathology are further addressed in different sections.

5.1 INTRODUCTION

In most cases chronic valvular lesions do not result in acute hemodynamic deterioration, although the patient with uncorrected end-stage aortic or mitral disease will eventually develop severe, irreducible heart failure. The overall clinical picture of acute severe mitral or aortic regurgitation is a variable combination of rapidly evolving shock and left ventricular (LV) failure, but occasional patients may tolerate them surprisingly well.

The acute valvular pathologies associated with possible new onset hemodynamic instability and their main common echocardiographic features are discussed below.

5.2 MAIN MECHANISMS FOR ACUTE VALVULAR REGURGITATION

- *Native valves*
  - ○ Acute mitral regurgitation (MR)
    - ■ Spontaneous chordae tendinae rupture
    - ■ Infectious endocarditis

A. Chenzbraun, *Emergency Echocardiography*, DOI: 10.1007/978-1-84882-336-5_5,
© Springer-Verlag London Limited 2009

- – leaflet perforation or disruption
- – chordal rupture
  - ■ Complicating an acute myocardial infarction (see Sect. 6.4)
  - ■ Traumatic (see Sect. 12.5)
- ○ Acute aortic regurgitation (AR)
  - ■ Infectious endocarditis
    - – leaflet perforation or disruption
  - ■ Type A aortic dissection
  - ■ Traumatic (see Sect. 12.5)
- • Prosthetic valves (see Sect. 12.2 and Appendix G)
  - ○ Mechanical valves
    - ■ Stuck valve
      - – Clot
      - – Pannus
      - – Vegetation
    - ■ Paravalvular leak
  - ○ Bioprosthetic valves
    - ■ Paravalvular leak
    - ■ Vegetation
    - ■ Degenerated valve

5.3 COMMON ECHOCARDIOGRAPHIC FINDINGS WITH ACUTE VALVULAR REGURGITATION

Acute valvular regurgitations result in acute ventricular volume overload, therefore my share some common features, irrespective of the specific valve involved:

- • Severe regurgitant jet (eccentric jets may be underevaluated)
- • Hyperdynamic LV* (in the absence of previous impairment)
- • Pulmonary hypertension, possibly enlarged and hypokinetic right ventricular (RV)
- • The specific pathology responsible**

The finding of a hyperdynamic ventricle in a patient who clinically is in severe acute cardiac failure should prompt a search for acute regurgitation.
**Not always obvious from a transthoracic study.*

5.4 SPECIFIC VALVULAR PATHOLOGIES

5.4.1 Native Valve Pathology: Acute MR

5.4.1.1 Acute MR Due to Spontaneous Chordal Rupture
Spontaneous chordal rupture is a possible complication of degenerative mitral valve disease, [1] that is, myxomatous degeneration

or fibroelastic deficiency. Frequently, these patients are diagnosed because of either a murmur or progressive heart failure symptoms. However, a small minority of previously healthy patients will present with a dramatic picture of pulmonary edema and, possibly, shock. Auscultatory findings may be unreliable in this context but a possible clinical clue to suspect the diagnosis is the acute onset of pulmonary edema in absence of any identifiable etiology. *Urgent echocardiography should always be performed with unexplained pulmonary edema.*

The overall echocardiographic picture will include (Fig. 5.1):

- Hyperdynamic ventricle
- Severe mitral regurgitant jet

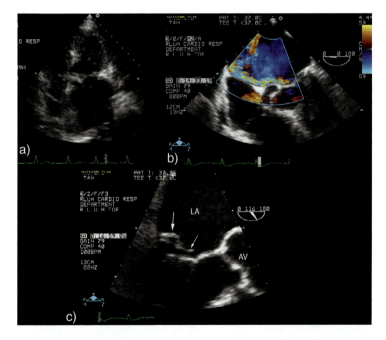

FIG. 5.1. Emergency echocardiography in a patient with sudden onset of unexplained acute pulmonary edema in whom transthoracic echocardiography (*TTE*) showed a hyperdynamic heart and possibly a very eccentric mitral regurgitation (*MR*) jet. **a** Transthoracic apical 4-chamber view showing small end systolic ventricular volume consistent with a hyperdynamic ventricle. **b** Transesophageal echocardiography (*TEE*) imaging at 0° in mid-esophageal position with clockwise rotation, confirms the diagnostic of severe MR with eccentric, anteriorly directed jet. **c** TEE scanning at 116° in mid-high esophageal position demonstrates flail central scallop of the posterior mitral leaflet (*thick arrow*) with ruptured chorda (*thin arrow*).

- ○ eccentric and, thus, possibly underestimated or even missed altogether *or*
- ○ extremely wide, completely filling the left atrium.
- The specific valvular pathology involved
  - ○ a torn chorda and/or a flail leaflet can be seen sometimes on a transthoracic echocardiography (TTE) but if in doubt or for better visualization, transesophageal echocardiography (TEE) is needed.
- Pulmonary hypertension and various degrees of right ventricular enlargement and failure

5.4.1.2 Acute MR Due to Infective Endocarditis

The mitral valve can be involved in infective endocarditis (IE) either primarily or due to extension from aortic valve endocarditis, so *the importance of careful scanning of all valves in IE patients cannot be overemphasized*. Acute MR can develop mainly as a result of:

- progressive leaflets destruction
- vegetation impeding the leaflets coaptation in systole
- localized leaflet perforation, and
- chordal rupture.

Especially with the last two mechanisms, the MR occurrence or worsening can be rapid and dramatic, translating clinically in pulmonary edema and shock. The echocardiographic findings will include the common findings of acute severe MR and specific changes as described above, though, occasionally, the degree of regurgitation will be unexpectedly milder than anticipated (Fig. 5.2).

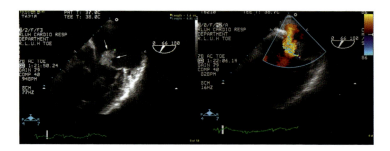

Fig. 5.2. Transesophageal echocardiography (*TEE*) study in a patient with staphylococcal infective endocarditis (*IE*). **a** Large vegetation is present on the atrial side of the leaflets. **b** Color Doppler shows mild-moderate mitral regurgitation (*MR*) only.

5.4.2   Native Valve Pathology: Acute AR

There are three instances of acute, hemodynamically compromising, aortic regurgitation (see below). Echocardiographically, they share the finding of a possibly hyperdynamic ventricle and the visualization of the wide and turbulent regurgitant jet by color Doppler. The specific findings will reflect the etiology.

5.4.2.1   Infective Endocarditis (Fig. 5.3)

The presence of vegetation and/or leaflet disruption/perforation should be seen on either TTE or TEE.

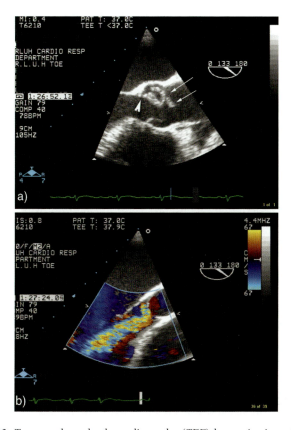

FIG. 5.3. Transesophageal echocardiography (*TEE*) long-axis view of aortic root in a patient with acute endocarditis and hemodynamic deterioration. **a** Thickened aortic non-coronary cusp with complex, elongated vegetation with a mobile part (*thin arrows*). A small area of valve disruption is seen at the base of the leaflet (*thick arrow*). **b** Diastolic frame in the same view with color Doppler demonstrates severe aortic regurgitation with eccentric jet.

5.4.2.2 Type A Aortic Dissection

Acute or worsening AR is frequently found in the setting of type A aortic dissection, due to:

- tethering of the leaflets by the dilated aortic root,
- change in the valvular geometry, and
- prolapse of intimal flap through the valve.

Though the presence of AR in these patients can generally be documented by TTE, TEE is necessary to clarify the mechanism involved.

5.4.2.3 Blunt Chest Trauma (See Sect. 12.5)

Aortic cusps disruption can rarely occur with severe chest trauma. This emphasizes the need for an echocardiographic scan in unstable patients after severe blunt chest trauma.

5.5 ACUTE PROSTHETIC VALVE PATHOLOGY (SEE ALSO SECT. 12.3 AND APPENDIX G)

There are five main pathological processes that may affect the functioning of prosthetic valves (Table 5.1). The resulting clinical entities and the echocardiographic diagnostic approach are discussed below.

5.5.1 Stuck Prosthetic Valve [2-4]

Represents acute or rapidly progressive limitation of the motion of the valve occluder (ball, disk, leaflets). Although, it is generally associated with obstruction, a stuck valve may become regurgitant if the closing excursion of the occluder is impeded as well.

Can occur in:

- Mechanical valves, due to:
  - Thrombus formation – more likely with
    - inadequate anticoagulation
    - shorter time interval from valve implantation.
  - Pannus (fibrous tissue) growth - more likely with:
    - long-time interval from valve implantation.
  - Vegetation
- Bioprosthetic valves, due to:
  - Vegetation

Risk factors for stuck valve include

- Mitral position
- Low cardiac output
- Atrial fibrillation

TABLE 5.1. Main pathologies involving mechanical and biological prosthetic valves.

| | Prosthetic valve type | | Clinical and echocardiographical picture | | | |
	Mechanical	Biological	Valvular obstruction	Valvular regurgitation	Paravalvular regurgitation	Embolism
Thrombosis[a]	+	−	+	+	−	+
Pannus[a]	+	−	+	+	−	−
Infection	+	+	+	+	+	+
"Wear and tear"[b]	−	+	+	+	+	−

[a]For all practical purposes, restriction of valve motion due to thrombus or pannus is a mechanical valve pathology
[b]"Wear and tear" deterioration of mechanical valves is not a practical concern anymore but it is a limiting factor for durability of bioprosthetic valves

The clinical picture will include:

- Rapidly progressing heart failure and/or hypotension up to shock and pulmonary edema
- Possible new murmur and/or muffling of prosthesis sounds

The echocardiographic workup of a suspected obstructed valve is detailed in Sect. 12.2.

5.5.2 Regurgitant Prosthetic Valve[5]

A prosthetic valve can become acutely regurgitant as part of a "stuck" condition, as detailed above, or due to a paravalvular leak. The progressive regurgitation due to "wear and tear" of a bioprosthetic valve is a more chronic process, so it will not be included in this discussion.

5.5.2.1 Paravalvular Leaks

Small (<5mm) dehiscences are not unusual in postmortem studies.[5] Clinically significant paravalvular leaks may result from failure of the sutures in prone areas, especially in patients with heavily calcified or degenerated valvular annuli, but are mainly the result of prosthetic valve endocarditis. From a practical standpoint, the acute development of a paravalvular leak should always prompt a workup to rule out infective endocarditis. Besides the possible signs and symptoms of endocarditis, the acute emergence of a significant paravalvular leak may manifest itself as a combination of:

- New murmur
- New onset/rapidly progressive cardiac failure
- Hemolytic anemia

Possible echocardiographic findings with severe paravalvular leaks are (Fig. 5.4):

- De novo hyperdynamic contractility
- High peak gradient with a normal mean gradient
  - *for a prosthetic valve in mitral position, a peak velocity of ≥2m/s with a normal (<5mmHg) mean gradient and a normal pressure half-time ($P_{1/2}T$) is highly suggestive of at least moderate regurgitation.*
- Visualization of a high velocity, turbulent jet, different from the normal appearance for a given valve
- "Rocking" motion of the valve if the dehiscence involves a large portion of the suture circumference

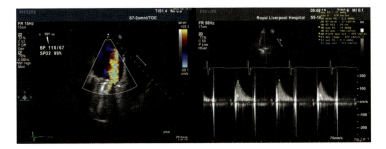

FIG. 5.4. Severe paravalvular leak in a patient with prosthetic mechanical valve in mitral position. **a** Transesophageal echocardiography (*TEE*) study showing a high velocity, turbulent regurgitant jet with a broad neck, originating between the mitral valve and the left atrium (*LA*) wall (*arrows*). **b** Transthoracic CW Doppler interrogation of the mitral flow revealing a high peak and a normal mean gradient.

Caveats in the echocardiographic assessment of suspected prosthetic valve regurgitation:

- Regurgitant mitral jets may be easily missed by TTE due to acoustic shadowing and require TEE for confident diagnosis
- In patients with aortic and mitral valve replacement, the aortic valve is frequently better assessed with TTE rather than with TEE, due to shadowing by the prosthetic mitral valve.

References

1. Hickey AJ, Wilcken DE, Wright JS, Warren BA. Primary (spontaneous) chordal rupture: relation to myxomatous valve disease and mitral valve prolapse. *J Am Coll Cardiol.* 1985;5(6):1341–1346.
2. Barbetseas J, Nagueh SF, Pitsavos C, Toutouzas PK, Quiñones MA, Zoghbi WA. Differentiating thrombus from pannus formation in obstructed mechanical prosthetic valves: an evaluation of clinical, transthoracic and transesophageal echocardiographic parameters. *J Am Coll Cardiol.* 1998;32(5):1410–1417.
3. Roudaut R, Roques X, Lafitte S, et al. Surgery for prosthetic valve obstruction. A single center study of 136 patients. *Eur J Cardiothorac Surg.* 2003;24(6):868–872.
4. Vitale N, Renzulli A, Agozzino L, et al. Obstruction of mechanical mitral prostheses: analysis of pathologic findings. *Ann Thorac Surg.* 1997:63(4):1101–1106.
5. Safi AM, Kwan T, Afflu E, Kamme AA, Salciccioli L. Paravalvular regurgitation: a rare complication following valve replacement surgery. *Angiology.* 2000;51(6):479–487.

Chapter 6
Echocardiography in Acute Chest Pain and Coronary Syndromes

Echocardiography is widely used in the assessment and management of acute coronary syndromes. This chapter covers various topics from risk stratification in the emergency room to the diagnosis of mechanical complications of acute myocardial infarction (AMI) such as acute mitral regurgitation (MR) and interventricular septum and free wall rupture. A special section is dedicated to the increasingly recognized occurrence of transient left ventricular outflow tract (LVOT) obstruction and MR in the setup of acute anterior myocardial infarction.

6.1 INTRODUCTION
In patients with acute chest pain or proven acute coronary syndromes (ACS), echocardiography is used with the following indications:

- Acute chest pain syndromes when ischemic etiology has to be confirmed or ruled out
- ACS where early assessment is needed for prompt management; this includes risk stratification, hemodynamic instability, and mechanical complications of AMI
- Predischarge evaluation after an acute coronary syndrome

Within the scope of this book, only the first two indications will be addressed.

A. Chenzbraun, *Emergency Echocardiography*, DOI: 10.1007/978-1-84882-336-5_6,
© Springer-Verlag London Limited 2009

6.2 ECHOCARDIOGRAPHY IN ACUTE CHEST PAIN SYNDROMES

Acute chest pain is a common presentation in emergency departments, yet an ischemic event is eventually confirmed in only a minority of these patients. Diagnostic and immediate risk stratification algorithms use clinical features, ECG changes and biochemical markers such as troponin, so a timely decision can be made whether to discharge or admit the patient with a view to further investigations. However, a combination of atypical symptoms on one side, high risk factors profile, and nonspecific ECG abnormalities on the other side may prove a diagnostic challenge. This can be rendered even more difficult by mildly elevated troponin levels in patients with renal failure. With the increasing demands on clinicians for faster triage and earlier discharge, additional tests for myocardial ischemia are necessary. In this context, echocardiography may be integrated in an accurate and cost-effective strategy for the rapid assessment of chest pain in an emergency department.

New or transient regional wall motion abnormalities are the echocardiographic hallmark of myocardial ischemia. LV assessment in the emergency department, eventually using a hand-held machine or including more advanced techniques such as stress echo and myocardial perfusion studies, has been thoroughly investigated. In these studies, echocardiography showed both good correlation and complementary diagnostic value with troponin levels and good predictive value.[1–5] Though a generally accepted strategy for the use of echocardiography in the rapid triage of patients with chest pain has yet to be agreed upon, *lack of new wall motion abnormalities identifies a low risk population of patients who, in the appropriate clinical context, may benefit of shorter observation periods or early discharge*. The liberal use of echocardiography in these patients can also assist the diagnosis of nonischemic cardiac pathology such as pericardial effusion or aortic dissection. The potential indications, limitations and caveats of this approach are detailed below.

6.2.1 Indications
- Lack of concordance between clinical presentation, ECG and ischemia markers
- Borderline or nondiagnostic ECG or biochemical ischemia markers
- Chest pain with hemodynamic instability

6.2.2 Advantages
- Diagnosis of borderline cases
- Additional information is obtained:

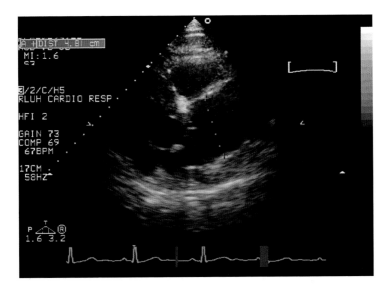

FIG. 6.1. Transthoracic parasternal long axis view in a young patient admitted with severe chest pain and nonspecific ECG changes. LV contractility was normal but there was significant dilatation of the aortic root and the aortic valve was bicuspid. The pain was interpreted as possible stretching or ongoing dilatation of the ascending aorta and the patient underwent aortic root replacement.

- ○ Severity (as reflected in the degree and extent of hypokinesis) and location (e.g., anterior vs posterior in the presence of anterior ST depression) of myocardial ischemia
- ○ Presence of important nonischemic pathology
  - ▪ Valvular pathology
  - ▪ Pericardial effusion
  - ▪ Aortic pathology (FIG. 6.1)

6.2.3   Limitations
- Good quality images and appropriate echocardiographic skills for accurate interpretation are an absolute must.
- Equipment and expertise logistical constraints may limit the widespread use of this approach.

6.2.4   Caveats
- In the absence of a previous echo study, a wall motion abnormality cannot be confidently diagnosed as new unless it is

shown to be dynamic; however, in a patient without any previous cardiac history it may be assumed to be new.

- With unstable angina as opposed to MI, a wall motion abnormality may be detected only if the scan is performed while the patient is experiencing pain.
- Mild ischemia in a small territory can be missed.

6.3 RISK STRATIFICATION AND EARLY ASSESSMENT

Early echocardiographic assessment is not routinely needed in uncomplicated ACS cases and strategies exist for echo-based pre-discharge evaluation. In ACS patients, echocardiography should be strongly considered at any time with the following:

6.3.1 Unclear Clinical Picture

- ACS cases with hemodynamic instability
  - ○ Look for:
    - □ Global and regional ventricular function
    - □ LV filling patterns
    - □ Unsuspected valvular pathology
    - □ Pericardial fluid
- Suspected right ventricular infarction (RVI) - In patients with inferior MI, RVI should be suspected with the occurrence of the following:
  - ○ Transient ST elevation in right precordial leads
  - ○ Persistent hypotension
  - ○ Exaggerated hypotensive response to nitrates
  - ○ Raised JVP without clear left sided heart failure findings
  - ○ Look for:
    - □ RV size and function
    - □ Tricuspid regurgitation
    - □ LV function and filling patterns
    - □ In hypoxaemic patients: PFO with right-to-left shunt due to increased right side pressures

6.3.2 Ongoing Ischemia

- Look for location and severity of wall motion abnormalities

6.3.3 *Ischemic Stroke or Peripheral Embolism*

Look for LV thrombus (LVT). LVT is generally associated with anterior MI and apical location (Fig. 6.2) but can occur with posterior or inferior MI as well. *With large infarctions, thrombus formation can occur as early as a few hours after onset.* If LVT is present, measure dimension by 2-D and assess:

- Location:

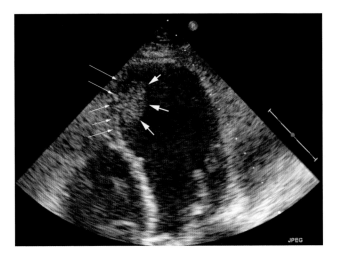

FIG. 6.2. Large, protruding, pedunculated thrombus (*thick arrows*) in patient with apical aneurysm. Note the thin, infarcted apical septum (*thin arrows*)

- ○ Generally, LVT develops in an aneurysmal area which has to be described in terms of site and size. Careful scanning is necessary in order not to miss the true apex due to foreshortening.
- Mobility
- Morphology:
  - ○ Mural
  - ○ Protruding

6.4 MECHANICAL COMPLICATIONS OF AMI

6.4.1 Acute MR in the Onset of AMI

Various degrees of echocardiographic MR are common in the acute and subacute phase of MI; however, moderate-severe MR is reported in just 6–13% and hemodynamically significant MR resulting in acute decompensation develops in a minority only.[6] With severe acute MR, the clinical picture can be dramatic with sudden hemodynamic deterioration, shock and pulmonary edema or with more insidious, but nevertheless rapidly developing, heart failure.

Understanding the underlying mechanism is crucial for a correct echocardiographic assessment with surgical implications.

The clinical characteristics, mechanisms, and echocardiographic findings of MR following an AMI are discussed below and summarized in Table 6.1.

TABLE 6.1. Clinical characteristics, echocardiographic findings and mechanisms of severe MR following an acute MI, listed by the time of onset.

	Dynamic LVOT obstruction	PM rupture	Localized MV distortion	Global LV remodeling
Timing	Hyperacute phase	Acute phase	Acute to subacute phase	Subacute to chronic phase
MI localization	Anterior	Inferior/posterior	Inferior/posterior	Anterior
MI size	Large	Small	Variable	Large
Hyperdynamic LV[a]	Basal segments only	Except inferior segment	Variable	No
Jet direction	Eccentric (posterior)	Eccentric (variable)	Eccentric (posterior)	Central
Specific findings	Systolic anterior motion of AML LVOT obstruction	Highly mobile mass in LA	Localized basal inferoposterior akinesis restricted PML motion	Apical displacement (tenting) of both leaflets

[a]The combination of acute pulmonary edema and hyperdynamic ventricle occurring a few days after an inferior MI is highly suggestive of acute MR and should prompt a TEE if the diagnosis is not established by TTE
AML: anterior mitral leaflet, LA: left atrium, PM: papillary muscle, PML: posterior mitral leaflet

6.4.1.1 Rupture of a Papillary Muscle

Though the most dramatic, this is not, however, the most frequent mechanism. Papillary muscle rupture is a rare (1%)[6] and serious complication of acute MI. It involves mainly the posterior papillary muscle which is vascularized by the RCA or the LCx only, rather than the anterior papillary muscle, which has a double vascular supply from both the RCA or the LCx and the LAD. Accordingly, papillary muscle rupture is more common with inferior MI. Total transection of the papillary muscle is usually a fatal event, while rupture of a head only may allow patient survival and time for intervention. Since the posterior papillary muscle supports both the posterior and the anterior mitral leaflets,[7] either the anterior or the posterior leaflets segments may be involved, with resulting severe eccentric MR.

Echocardiographic features (Fig. 6.3):

• Hyperdynamic LV with the possible exception of the basal inferior or posterior wall and evidence of pulmonary hypertension with some degree of RV enlargement and decreased contractility are common.

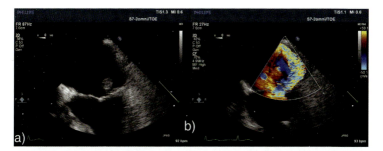

FIG. 6.3. Transesophageal scanning at 0° in mid-esophageal position in a patient admitted with a small inferior MI and who developed acute pulmonary edema with a hyperdynamic ventricle. **a** 2D imaging shows intact mitral leaflets and a highly mobile rounded mass in the left atrium representing a ruptured papillary muscle head. **b** Color Doppler demonstrates a wide MR jet, directed posteriorly, indicating anterior mitral leaflet pathology. At surgery, partial posterior papillary muscle rupture was confirmed involving the chordae supporting the A3 segment of the anterior mitral leaflet.

- Eccentric regurgitant jet, directed either anteriorly or posteriorly depending on the leaflet involved.
- *The patognomonic finding is the presence of a highly mobile mass in the left atrium, prolapsing from the LV in every systole.*
- Usually the diagnosis is evident on a TTE study, though, occasionally, TEE is necessary.

6.4.1.2 Altered Local Geometry of the Mitral Apparatus

Inferior/posterior MI can induce severe MR by retraction of the papillary muscle and local remodeling of the basal posterior wall. Subsequent valve tethering and asymmetrical posterior annular dilatation result in malcoaptation and eccentric regurgitation. The clinical picture is of rapidly developing cardiac failure soon after an inferior/posterior MI.

Echocardiographic features (Fig. 6.4):

- Evidence of inferior/posterior MI with hypercontractility of noninfarcted segments
- Eccentric, posteriorly oriented jet[*]
- Restricted posterior mitral leaflet with relative prolapse of the AML which 'slides' against the posterior leaflet.[**]

[*]Note that the jet has the same orientation as in Fig. 6.3 though the mechanisms involved are different.

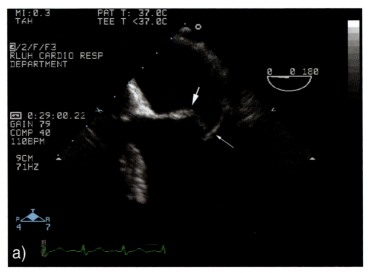

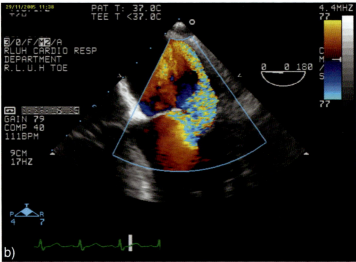

FIG. 6.4. Transesophageal scanning at 0° in mid-esophageal position in a patient admitted with a large infero-posterior MI who developed rapidly progressive cardiac failure during hospitalization. **a** 2D imaging showing a restricted posterior leaflet (*thin arrow*) which fails to reach the annular plane. The anterior leaflet (*thick arrow*) does not ascend above the annular plane but relative prolapse and lack of coaptation occur nevertheless. **b** Color Doppler demonstrates severe MR with eccentric jet.

**The mitral apparatus may appear deceptively normal in some patients and the clue to the mechanism is the posteriorly oriented jet of severe MR in the setup of recent inferior MI.

6.4.1.3 General Distortion of the Mitral Apparatus

The chronic phase of large anterior infarctions is characterized by global ventricular remodeling with the left ventricle becoming bigger and assuming a more spherical shape. This results in mitral annulus dilatation and apical tethering of both leaflets in a manner similar to that encountered in nonischemic cardiomyopathies.[8] As a consequence, coaptation at annular level is prevented and severe, central MR can occur (Fig. 6.5). This is a more chronic and evolving process which generally does not result in acute regurgitation. However, it can develop rapidly in cases with extensive anterior MI and early remodeling.

6.4.1.4 Systolic Anterior Motion of the Mitral Valve with Dynamic LVOT Obstruction

This is a special and rare kind of transient MR occurring in the hyperacute phase of MI. It is discussed in Sect. 6.4.4.

6.4.2 Acute Ventricular Septal Rupture

Acute septal rupture is an uncommon and serious complication of MI, occurring generally in the first few days after the acute event. The advent of thrombolysis markedly reduced the incidence of AVSR from 1–3% to less than 0.5%, though the onset tends to be earlier in thrombolysed cases.[9] Septal rupture is associated more frequently with anterior MI, but is definitely possible with inferior MI as well. With anterior MI the defect is generally located in the apical septum, while with inferior MI it involves the basal inferior septum. The typical clinical picture is of acute hemodynamic deterioration and appearance of a new, harsh systolic murmur. Either septal rupture or acute MR has to be considered with this clinical scenario. Historically, Swan–Ganz catheterization was used to confirm a step-up in saturations at RV level, but presently, AVSR diagnosis is essentially an echocardiographic one. The rupture is identified by color Doppler which will show a high velocity, turbulent jet entering the right ventricle (Fig. 6.6). Careful scanning should clarify the ventricular septal defect (VSD) location. For surgical planning, besides confirming the VSD and its position, the echocardiographic report should specifically include:

- Overall LV contractility
- Presence or absence of an aneurysm
- RV size and function
- Presence and severity of pulmonary hypertension

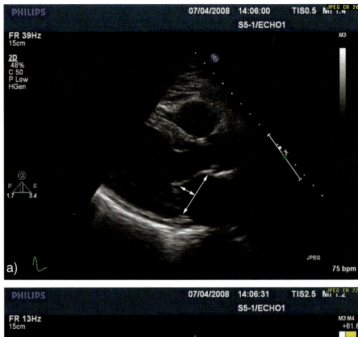

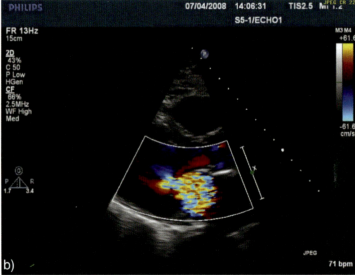

FIG. 6.5. Systolic frame in PSLA view in a patient with a recent large anterior MI and severely decreased LV function. **a** 2D image shows the two mitral leaflets tethered apically and coapting at a distance (*short arrow*) from the annular plane (*long arrow*). **b** Color Doppler demonstrates severe MR with a central jet.

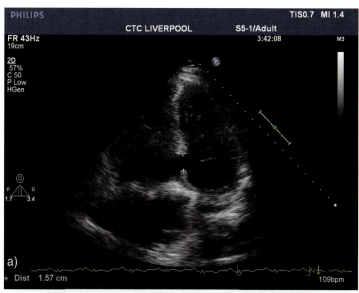

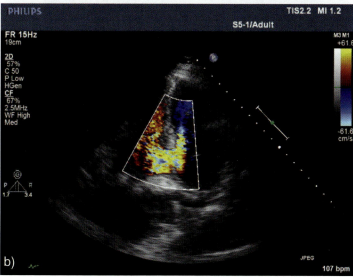

FIG. 6.6. Large basal inferior septum ventricular septal rupture in a patient with an inferior MI. **a** 2D imaging in apical 4-chamber view reveals the lack of tissue continuity (*small crosses*) at base of the septum. Note the dilated RV, secondary to acute right ventricle overload. **b** Color Doppler reveals the wide turbulent jet across the defect, consistent with a large left-to-right shunt.

6.4.3 Acute and Subacute Free Wall Rupture

Acute free rupture is a catastrophic and usually fatal event with the patient rapidly developing cardiogenic shock and pulseless electrical activity unresponsive to resuscitation. If the rupture is small, or with a serpiginous path, the slower accumulation of blood in the pericardial cavity may allow time for diagnosis and emergency intervention (subacute rupture). A sudden reoccurrence of pain, possibly with ST re-elevation and rapid hemodynamic deterioration with tamponade features should raise the suspicion of free wall rupture. Emergency echocardiography is mandatory with this clinical scenario. The presence of pericardial fluid >5 mm in this context supports the diagnosis, especially if a dense intrapericardial mass consistent with clot is visualized[10,11] (Fig. 6.7).

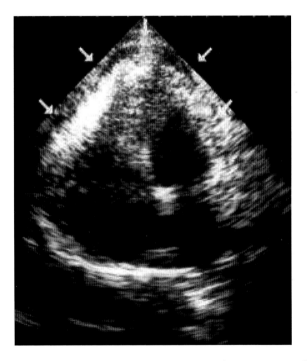

FIG. 6.7. 2D apical 4-chamber view in a patient with acute MI complicated by subacute free wall rupture. A small pericardial effusion is noted around the apex (*arrows*) and a thick, dense echogenic mass overlies the RV free wall. (Reproduced from Raposo et al.,[11] open publication policy).

Of note, *the finding of pericardial fluid as such, without the typical clinical picture is not diagnostic of cardiac rupture since small amounts are not infrequent with AMI.*

6.4.4 Acute Dynamic MR and LVOT Obstruction

Patients with large apical infarctions and hyperdynamic base of the heart can develop in the hyperacute phase systolic anterior motion of the mitral valve (SAM) with resulting severe MR and left ventricular outflow tract (LVOT) obstruction. The clinical suspicion should be raised by the development of severe MR in the first hours of a large anterior MI, as opposed to the typical acute MR which has a later onset and is more common with inferior MI. SAM and LVOT obstruction should be actively sought in these cases since the management is quite specific including beta blockers and avoidance of vasodilators. This complication is reported in the literature,[12,13] though it is still not included in the formal list of mechanical complications of acute MI. These patients tend to have single LAD disease and some degree of basal septal hypertrophy or have the transient apical ballooning described as Takotsubo cardiomyopathy in patients with normal coronary arteries who present with a clinical and ECG picture mimicking a large anterior MI (see Sect. 12.1.2).

References

1. Autore C, Agati L, Piccininno M, Lino S, Musaro S. Role of echocardiography in acute chest pain syndrome. *Am J Cardiol*. 2000;86(4A):41G–42G.
2. Bholasingh R, Cornel JH, Kamp O, et al. Prognostic value of predischarge dobutamine stress echocardiography in chest pain patients with a negative cardiac troponin T. *J Am Coll Cardiol*. 2003;41(4):596–602.
3. Buchsbaum M, Marshall E, Levine B, et al. Emergency department evaluation of chest pain using exercise stress echocardiography. *Acad Emerg Med*. 2001;8(2):196–199.
4. Mohler ER 3rd, Ryan T, Segar SD, et al. Clinical utility of troponin T levels and echocardiography in the emergency department. *Am Heart J*. 1998;135(2 Pt 1):253–260.
5. Weston P, Alexander JH, Patel MR, Maynard C, Crawford L, Wagner GS. Hand-held echocardiographic examination of patients with symptoms of acute coronary syndromes in the emergency department: the 30-day outcome associated with normal left ventricular wall motion. *Am Heart J*. 2004;148(6):1096–1101.
6. Birnbaum Y, Chamoun AJ, Conti VR, et al. Mitral regurgitation following acute myocardial infarction. *Coron Artery Dis*. 2002;13(6):337–344.

7. Ho SY. Anatomy of the mitral valve. *Heart*. 2002;88(Suppl 4):iv5–iv10.
8. Levine RA, Schwammenthal E. Ischemic mitral regurgitation on the threshold of a solution: from paradoxes to unifying concepts. *Circulation*. 2005;112(5):745–758.
9. Birnbaum Y, Fishbein MC, Blanche C, Siegel RJ. Ventricular septal rupture after acute myocardial infarction. *N Engl J Med*. 2002;347(18):1426–1432.
10. Lopez-Sendon J, Gonzales A, Lopez S, et al. Diagnosis of subacute ventricular wall rupture after acute myocardial infarction: sensitivity and specificity of clinical, hemodynamic and echocardiographic criteria. *J Am Coll Cardiol*. 1992;19(6):1145–1153.
11. Raposo L, Andrade MJ, Ferreira J, et al. Subacute left ventricle free wall rupture after acute myocardial infarction: awareness of the clinical signs and early use of echocardiography may be life-saving. *Cardiovasc Ultrasound*. 2006;4:46.
12. Chockalingam A, Tejwani L, Aggarwal K, et al. Dynamic left ventricular outflow tract obstruction in acute myocardial infarction with shock: cause, effect, and coincidence. *Circulation*. 2007;116(5):e110–e113.
13. Hrovatin E, Piazza R, Pavan D, et al. Dynamic left ventricular outflow tract obstruction in the setting of acute anterior myocardial infarction: a serious and potentially fatal complication? *Echocardiography*. 2002;19(6):449–455.

Chapter 7
Echocardiography in Acute Aortic Syndromes

This chapter covers the excellent diagnostic capabilities and the few limitations of transesophageal echocardiography in the diagnosis of the three presentations of acute aortic syndromes: aortic dissection (AD), intramural hematoma (IMH), and penetrating aortic ulcer (PAU). An algorithm for deciding on the appropriate imaging strategy in patients with suspected acute aortic syndromes is included, as well as a listing of echocardiographic information to be actively sought when assessing a patient with acute aortic dissection.

7.1 INTRODUCTION
Aortic syndromes are a group of conditions characterized by symptoms suggestive of acute aortic pathology and subsequent diagnosis of AD, IMH, or PAU.

7.2 AORTIC DISSECTION
AD is a major emergency with a 1–2% hourly mortality in the first 48 h, without appropriate treatment. The clinical presentation, and the diagnostic and therapeutic approaches, are well described[1–3]; in intensive care units (ICU) patients, where symptoms are less reliable, a combination of newly enlarged mediastinum on chest X-rays, hemodynamic instability, stroke, peripheral, or visceral ischemia syndrome should raise the suspicion of AD. For practical purposes, a convenient classification is the Stanford classification, whereby all dissections involving the ascending aorta are type A and all dissections where the

A. Chenzbraun, *Emergency Echocardiography*, DOI: 10.1007/978-1-84882-336-5_7,
© Springer-Verlag London Limited 2009

De Bakey Classification

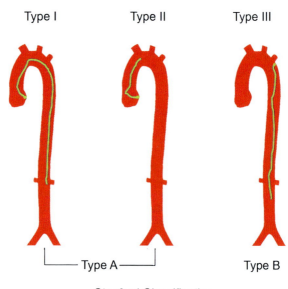

Type I   Type II   Type III

Type A   Type B

Stanford Classification

FIG. 7.1. The two widely used classification systems of thoracic aortic dissection. The Stanford one relates only to the involvement or sparing of the ascending aorta, while the De Bakey system also distinguishes between dissections confined to the aortic root or extending more distally. Both type I and II in De Bakey classification would be assigned to type A by Stanford classification (yellow line: intimal flap).

ascending aorta is spared are type B,[4] (Fig. 7.1). Noninvasive techniques such as echocardiography, computed tomography (CT), and magnetic resonance imaging (MRI) have replaced aortography as diagnostic method of choice. Transesophageal echocardiography has excellent sensitivity and specificity for both type A (96% and 86%, respectively) and type B aortic dissection (100% and 96%, respectively), thus having a diagnostic accuracy comparable with that of CT and MRI and even transthoracic echocardiography (TTE) fares very well for type A aortic dissection.[5] Each medical institution should have an imaging protocol in place for the diagnosis of suspected AD. Which imaging modality is decided upon for a first line approach will necessarily reflect local resources and expertise. While MRI may offer the best sensitivity/specificity balance for all kinds of dissections, it is neither always available nor is suitable for acutely ill, unstable patients or for patients with mechanical implants. Some of these limitations hold true for CT as well, which in any case *has to be completed by at least a TTE scan to assess ventricular function and severity and mechanism of aortic regurgitation, if present*. TEE provides a rapid, bedside available, comprehensive diagnosis and is the method of choice when the need for diagnosis is urgent or if the patient is unstable. The safety of TEE in acute AD is excellent. Care should be taken that the patient is appropriately sedated and beta blocked for the procedure to avoid discomfort and possible raise in blood pressure. In stable patients, a combination of two imaging modalities, for example TTE and spiral CT, may be used. By definition, the echocardiographic diagnosis of dissection requires the visualization of the true and false lumen separated by the intimal flap. In some instances, the intimal flap has a typical presentation of a linear echo across the aortic lumen (Fig. 7.2) but, occasionally, its appearance may be puzzling to the

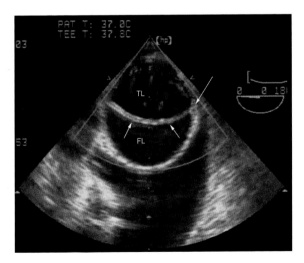

FIG. 7.2. Transesophageal scan in a patient with type B aortic dissection. Descending aorta is visualized at 0° with the scope rotated posteriorly in mid-esophageal position. A thick linear echo (*short arrows*) demonstrates the intimal flap separating the true lumen with evidence of flow by color Doppler and the false lumen, which has no flow. A small turbulent flow at 3 o'clock (*long arrow*) reveals the site of an intimal tear. The black, triangular space posterior to the aorta represents left pleural effusion. *FL* false lumen, *TL* true lumen.

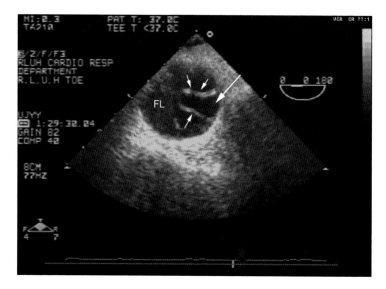

Fig. 7.3. Type B aortic dissection with a less common appearance of the flap (*short arrows*) encircling a compressed true lumen (*long arrow*). Increased echogenicity in the false lumen reflects blood stagnation.

inexperienced eye (Fig. 7.3). Also, linear artifacts may mimic a dissection flap, especially in the ascending aorta. The main limitation of TEE in this context is the presence of a "blind spot," due to tracheal and bronchial interposition, which interferes with visualization of the distal ascending aorta and proximal arch. The echocardiographic assessment of AD patients is an elaborate one and is not limited to recognizing or ruling out the intimal flap. *As such, TEE assessment of AD should be the provision of an experienced echocardiographer.* Essential information to be actively sought and reported includes

• Proximal and distal extent of dissection
• Number and location of intimal tears and amount of communicating flow between the two lumina
• Degree of spontaneous contrast in the false lumen (generally, the false lumen is larger and has lower velocity or no flow as compared with the true lumen which has a brisker flow and is more pulsatile)
• Involvement of neck vessels and coronary arteries
• Severity and mechanism of aortic regurgitation

- Ventricular function
- Presence of pericardial, pleural, and mediastinal fluid*

*A pleural effusion can develop as part of a local inflammatory reaction; however, the presence of fluid can signal bleeding and imminence of rupture and as such is an ominous finding prompting emergency intervention.

7.3   INTRAMURAL HEMATOMA

Intramural hematoma is considered to represent a variant of classical AD, possibly a stage in the development of full-fledged dissection. It has been described in 10–30% of patients with suspected AD.[2] Pathologically, it is an intramedial bleeding, which did not progress to intimal flap formation and delineation of a true and false lumen. In terms of symptoms, the clinical presentation is similar to that of a typical dissection though evidence of visceral or peripheral ischemia may be less frequent. The prognosis and management are similar to those of completed dissection to which it can evolve in about one-third of cases.[2] The echocardiographic diagnosis requires demonstration of a crescentic or circular grossly thickened (>7 mm) aortic wall, frequently with an

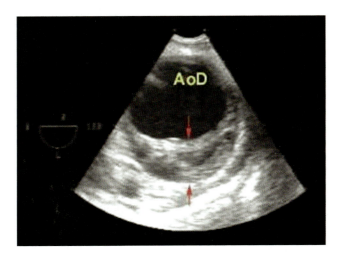

FIG. 7.4. Aortic intramural hematoma in the descending aorta. Note the semilunar massive thickening (arrows) of the posterior aortic wall and the echolucent zone between 5 and 6 o'clock. Reproduced with permission from Evangelista et al.[6]

intramural echolucent zone[6] (Fig. 7.4). The diagnosis of IMH as opposed to severe atherosclerotic plaque is supported by demonstrating the intimal layer overlying the abnormal area rather than being underneath but the differentiation from a severely diseased atherosclerotic aortic wall may be difficult.[7] An even greater challenge may be the differentiation from the thrombosed false lumen of a dissection without a detectable intimal tear, though in this case a misdiagnosis is less critical since the treatment is dictated by the localization of the aortic process and not by differentiating between the two entities.

7.4 PENETRATING AORTIC ULCER

Penetrating aortic ulcer is the result of an atherosclerotic ulceration disrupting the internal elastic lamina and advancing through the media with possible involvement of the full aortic wall thickness. The clinical presentation may be similar to that of a typical dissection and the process can develop to full-pledged dissection, IMH, pseudoaneurysm formation, or rupture and, in fact, these pathologies can coexist in the same patient.[8] Since PAU is strongly associated with aortic atherosclerosis, it involves mainly the descending aorta where severe atherosclerotic disease is more likely. The typical appearance of a penetrating ulcer is described as an outpouching of the aortic wall, generally associated with complex atherosclerotic wall changes.[8] The optimal management of PAU is still to be defined but recent reports suggest a good outcome using endovascular stent grafting.[9,10]

References

1. Januzzi JL, Isselbacher EM, Cooper JV, et al. Characterizing the young patient with aortic dissection: results from the International Registry of Aortic Dissection (IRAD). *J Am Coll Cardiol*. 2004;43(4):665-669.
2. Erbel R, Alfonso F, Boileau C, et al. Diagnosis and management of aortic dissection. *Eur Heart J*. 2001;22(18):1642-1681.
3. Ince H, Nienaber CA. Diagnosis and management of patients with aortic dissection. *Heart*. 2007;93(2):266–270.
4. Nienaber CA, Eagle KA. Aortic dissection: new frontiers in diagnosis and management: part I: from etiology to diagnostic strategies. *Circulation*. 2003;108(5):628–635.
5. Nienaber CA, von Kodolitsch Y, Nicolas V, et al. The diagnosis of thoracic aortic dissection by noninvasive imaging procedures. *N Engl J Med*. 1993;328(1):1–9.
6. Evangelista A, Avegliano G, Elorz C, González-Alujas T, del Castillo HG, Soler-Soler J. Transesophageal echocardiography in the diagnosis of acute aortic syndrome. *J Card Surg*. 2002;17(2):95–106.
7. Flachskampf FA. Assessment of aortic dissection and hematoma. *Semin Cardiothorac Vasc Anesth*. 2006;10(1):83–88.

8. Vilacosta I, San Roman JA, Aragoncillo P et al. Penetrating atherosclerotic aortic ulcer: documentation by transesophageal echocardiography. *J Am Coll Cardiol*. 1998;32(1):83–89.

9. Pauls S, Orend KH, Sunder-Plassmann L., Kick J, Schelzig, H et al. Endovascular repair of symptomatic penetrating atherosclerotic ulcer of the thoracic aorta. *Eur J Vasc Endovasc Surg*. 2007;34(1):66–73.

10. Botta L, Buttazzi K, Russo V et al. Endovascular repair for penetrating atherosclerotic ulcers of the descending thoracic aorta: early and mid-term results. *Ann Thorac Surg*. 2008;85(3):987–992.

Chapter 8
Echocardiography in Acute Pulmonary Embolism

High-risk pulmonary embolism (PE) is associated with significant right ventricular dilatation and hypocontractility. Major PE can be safely ruled out as a cause of hemodynamic deterioration if the right ventricle appears normal on a bedside echocardiographic study. This chapter details the role of emergency echocardiography in the diagnosis of patients with suspected PE, including the possible visualization of the thrombus with transesophageal echocardiography.

8.1 INTRODUCTION

PE is suspected whenever a patient presents with chest pain, dyspnea, hypoxemia, suggestive ECG changes, and an elevated D-dimer. Right ventricular failure and hemodynamic compromise define massive or high-risk PE while evidence of right ventricular (RV) impairment without hemodynamic instability define nonmassive or intermediate-risk PE.[1] Echocardiography is potentially useful in all cases but it has a special role in high- and intermediate-risk PE. These patients may be acutely ill with hypoxemia and cardiogenic shock and emergent echocardiography may strongly support the diagnosis of massive PE or make it unlikely. As a general rule, massive PE should cause significantly enough right ventricular enlargement and systolic dysfunction to be easily recognized on echocardiography (Fig. 8.1). Conversely, the absence of these findings practically rules out PE as the cause for the patient's hemodynamic deterioration.

A. Chenzbraun, *Emergency Echocardiography*, DOI: 10.1007/978-1-84882-336-5_8,
© Springer-Verlag London Limited 2009

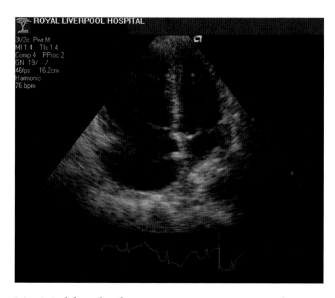

FIG. 8.1. Apical four-chamber view imaging in a patient with acute onset of chest pain, hypoxemia, and hypotension. There is severe dilatation and hypokinesis of the right ventricle and the interventricular septum is displaced toward an underfilled left ventricle. Massive pulmonary embolism (*PE*) was subsequently confirmed by computed tomography (*CT*) angiography.

Positive findings to be actively sought and reported in suspected massive PE are:
- RV enlargement and hypocontractility[*]
- Pulmonary artery dilatation
- Tricuspid regurgitation
- Dilated interior vena cava (IVC) with reduced respiratory varia tions
- Evidence for pulmonary hypertension[**]
  - As demonstrated by tricuspid regurgitation (TR) peak systolic velocity
  - As inferred by systolic flattening of the interventricular septum

[*]*The differential diagnosis between preexistent RV hypokinesis due to chronic lung disease and acutely developed RV failure due to PE may be occasionally challenging. Among others, preserved normal contractility of the RV apex in the presence of hypokinesis of the other RV free wall segments (McConell sign) has been reported as specific for the acute cor pulmonale, secondary to PE.[1]*

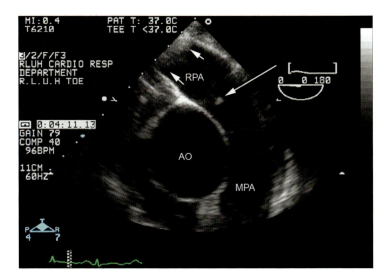

Fig. 8.2. Emergency transesophageal echocardiography (*TEE*) imaging of the pulmonary artery (*PA*) in a patient with evidence of a right atrial mass on transthoracic echocardiography (*TTE*), who became acutely hypoxemic. A small thrombus (*long arrow*) is seen at the origin of the right pulmonary artery, which more distally is almost totally obstructed by a large thrombus (*short arrows*). Computed tomography (*CT*) angiography confirmed multiple pulmonary emboli.

**The pulmonary artery (PA) pressure may be only moderately elevated with systemic hypotension and acute RV failure. PA pressure to systemic pressure ratio and IVS flattening may be more useful and demonstrate relative pulmonary hypertension even with relatively low TR velocities.

There is no practical role for echocardiography in the immediate diagnosis of suspected low-risk PE.

Though CT angiography is classically used to demonstrate PE, TEE is, again, a convenient alternative in critically ill patients who need a rapid, bedside diagnosis. The main PA, its bifurcation, and the right PA are easily visualized in most patients (Fig. 2.4c, 8.2). Since massive PE is frequently associated with either bilateral or main PA emboli, TEE should be able to visualize the obstructing embolus in these patients and indeed sensitivity and specificity of 80% and 100%, respectively, have been reported in severe PE.[2] Accordingly, TEE may be considered as a valid imaging method in critically ill patients with suspected massive PE allowing a rapid diagnostic confirmation.[3]

References

1. Torbicki A, Perrier A, Konstantinides S, et al. Guidelines on the diagnosis and management of acute pulmonary embolism: the task force for the diagnosis and management of acute pulmonary embolism of the European Society of Cardiology (ESC). *Eur Heart J.* 2008;29(18):2276–2315.
2. Pruszczyk P, Torbicki A, Pacho R, et al.. Noninvasive diagnosis of suspected severe pulmonary embolism: transesophageal echocardiography vs spiral CT. *Chest* 1997;112(3):722–728.
3. Krivec B, Voga G, Zuran I, et al. Diagnosis and treatment of shock due to massive pulmonary embolism: approach with transesophageal echocardiography and intrapulmonary thrombolysis. *Chest* 1997;112(5):1310–1316.

Chapter 9
Echocardiography in Stroke and Systemic Embolism

This chapter covers the main pathologies associated with stroke or a peripheral embolic event in acutely ill patients, with implications for an echocardiographic diagnosis.

Generally accepted algorithms are in place for the use of echocardiography in the work up of patients after an ischemic stroke or a peripheral embolism.[12] Depending on the overall clinical picture, the occurrence of an embolic event in a critically ill patient raises some specific diagnostic questions as detailed below.

- Left ventricular (LV) thrombus in a patient with acute/recent myocardial infarction
  - More likely with apical MI (Fig. 6.2)
- Left atrial thrombus in a patient with atrial fibrillation (Fig. 9.1)
  - More likely with mitral valve disease or LV dysfunction
- Native or prosthetic valve endocarditis
- Prosthetic valve thrombosis
- Aortic dissection
  - The tributary artery feeds from the false lumen

All these conditions *are echocardiographic diagnoses* so echocardiography should be used liberally in this clinical setup or if the presenting event is a systemic embolus, which, due to the size necessary to obstruct a peripheral or visceral artery is likely to be cardiac in origin.

A. Chenzbraun, *Emergency Echocardiography*, DOI: 10.1007/978-1-84882-336-5_9,
© Springer-Verlag London Limited 2009

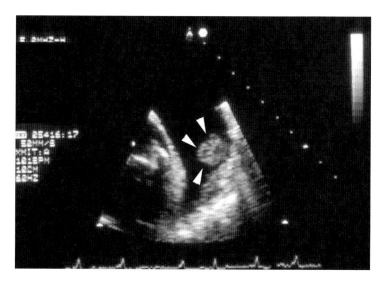

FIG. 9.1. Rounded, protruding thrombus (*arrow heads*) in a large left atrial appendage in a patient with atrial fibrillation.

References

1. Cheitlin MD, Alpert JS, Armstrong WF, et al. ACC/AHA guidelines for the clinical application of echocardiography: executive summary. A report of the American College of Cardiology/American Heart Association Task Force on Practice Guidelines (Committee on Clinical Application of Echocardiography). Developed in collaboration with the American Society of Echocardiography. *J Am Coll Cardiol*. 1997;29(4):862–879.
2. Douglas PS, Khandheria B, Stainback RF, et al. ACCF/ASE/ACEP/ ASNC/SCAI/SCCT/SCMR 2007 appropriateness criteria for tran- sthoracic and transesophageal echocardiography: a report of the American College of Cardiology Foundation Quality Strategic Directions Committee Appropriateness Criteria Working Group, American Society of Echocardiography, American College of Emergency Physicians, American Society of Nuclear Cardiology, Society for Cardiovascular Angiography and Interventions, Society of Cardiovascular Computed Tomography, and the Society for Cardiovascular Magnetic Resonance endorsed by the American College of Chest Physicians and the Society of Critical Care Medicine. *J Am Coll Cardiol*. 2007;50(2):187–204.

Chapter 10
Echocardiography in the Septic Patient

Maintenance of cardiac output may be compromised in sepsis due to a combination of myocardial depression and inappropriate vasodilatation. Echocardiographic information on both ventricular contractility and filling status is paramount for appropriate management. This chapter summarizes the role of echocardiography as an increasingly accepted alternative to invasive hemodynamic monitoring in septic patients.

Sepsis is diagnosed when there is evidence of both an infectious process and a systemic inflammatory response syndrome. The cardiovascular response to sepsis is complex and multifactorial, related to endothelial and coagulation system activation, microvascular dysfunction and release of numerous mediators, some of which, such as cytokines and prostanoids, act as myocardial depressors.[1] The hemodynamic hallmarks of sepsis are myocardial depression, which can range from occult to frank pump failure and inappropriate peripheral vasodilatation, which induces a hyperdynamic state and thus can mask mild degrees of myocardial dysfunction. *The majority of septic-shock patients will be hyperdynamic and vasodilated and benefit from fluid resuscitation and vasoconstrictors such as norepinephrine or dopamine*. A sizable minority of about one-third of the cases[2,3] can present nevertheless with decreased cardiac index and evidence of reduced ejection fraction and will require inotropic support with dobutamine as well.

Echocardiography in this setup can be performed as either a transthoracic or a transesophageal study depending on images quality and the existence of a specific indication for transesophageal

A. Chenzbraun, *Emergency Echocardiography*, DOI: 10.1007/978-1-84882-336-5_10,
© Springer-Verlag London Limited 2009

echocardiography (TEE). The main objectives of echocardiographic evaluation in the septic patient and the relevant echo findings to be specifically sought are:

- Confirmation of a hyperdynamic state and low filling pressures (see Sect. 3.3 and Fig. 3.2).
  - Hyperdynamic contraction of both ventricles; this is a subjective assessment, which, however, should be within the competence of even less-experienced operators.
  - E/A <1 and/or E/E' <10 by Doppler interrogation of the mitral valve and annulus are:
    - less useful with tachycardia when fusion of the early- and late-diastolic waves can occur.
  - Optional: actual measurement of cardiac index using the velocity time integral of the aortic flow and the aortic diameter (Appendix B)
- Prediction of response to fluid challenge:
  - >50% respiratory changes in inferior vena cava diameter
  - >60% respiratory changes in superior vena cava diameter (use TEE in ventilated patients)
- Exclusion/assessment of concomitant obvious systolic dysfunction.
- Unmasking of previously unrecognized left ventricular (LV) systolic dysfunction when the systemic vascular resistance is increased by using vasopressors. This requires a protocol of echocardiographic monitoring and may help to decide putting the patient on dobutamine as well.
- Confirmation or exclusion of possible endocarditis, when there are reasonable grounds to suspect this diagnosis.

The hemodynamic information input of echocardiography in these patients is of such quality and reliability that it should be seen as a viable alternative to invasive monitoring. In fact, some units report using repeat echo assessment as only mean of monitoring their septic patients.[3]

References

1. Merx MW, Weber C. Sepsis and the heart. *Circulation* 2007;116(7): 793–802.
2. Jardin F, Brun-Ney D, Auvert B, et al. Sepsis-related cardiogenic shock. *Crit Care Med.* 1990;18(10):1055–1060.
3. Vieillard-Baron A, Prin S, Chergui K, et al. Hemodynamic instability in sepsis: bedside assessment by Doppler echocardiography. *Am J Respir Crit Care Med.* 2003;168(11):1270–1276.

Chapter 11
Echocardiography During and After Resuscitation

Targeted echocardiography with a hand-held or portable device can provide vital information during cardiopulmonary resuscitation (CPR). This chapter addresses the role of echocardiography in identifying immediately treatable causes of pulseless electrical activity (PEA) and suggests an algorithm for emergency echocardiographic evaluation to be performed during advanced life support. Guidelines are also provided for echocardiographic studies in survivors, with an emphasis on the possibly transient nature of left ventricular dysfunction after resuscitation.

11.1   ECHOCARDIOGRAPHY-ASSISTED CPR

Echocardiography has been used in several resuscitation studies for either a better understanding of the hemodynamics or to clarify the diagnosis and optimize the procedure itself.[1-4] Also, the total absence of any cardiac mechanical activity visualized by echo, as opposed to the absence of a palpable peripheral pulse, portends an extremely poor prognosis and, thus, could be used in the decision-making process about cessation of resuscitative efforts.[5,6] The greatest potential role for echocardiography resides, however, in the immediate management of cardiac arrest with PEA. PEA has a much poorer prognosis than arrhythmic cardiac arrest [7-9] since it reflects either the terminal phase of pump failure such as following a massive infarction or is related to a major mechanical event which is not reversible unless specifically treated.

A. Chenzbraun, *Emergency Echocardiography*, DOI: 10.1007/978-1-84882-336-5_11,
© Springer-Verlag London Limited 2009

11.2 MECHANICAL EVENTS POTENTIALLY ASSOCIATED WITH PEA

11.2.1 Pulmonary Embolism (see Sect. 8)

- A severely dilated right ventricle (RV) with a normal or small left ventricle (LV) in a PEA patient is for any practical purpose diagnostic of massive pulmonary embolism

11.2.2 Tamponade (see Sect. 3.5)

- The presence of more than mild pericardial effusion with rather small ventricular cavities should be considered evidence of tamponade in a PEA patient
- Acute tamponade leading to PEA is more likely to be iatrogenic or posttraumatic rather than due to a medical condition, so confirmation of trauma or recent procedure should be sought

11.2.3 Hypovolemia (see Sect. 3.3)

A combination of the following in a PEA patient should raise a strong suspicion of severe acute hypovolemia (e.g., due to ruptured aortic aneurysm or any other massive internal bleeding)

- Small ventricular cavities with close opposite ventricular walls
- Collapsed (<5 mm diameter) interior vena cava (IVC)
- Hyperdynamic heart

11.2.4 Tension Pneumothorax

Should be suspected in the PEA patient with neck veins engorgement, especially after chest trauma or attempted central vein cannulation, when emergency echocardiography does not confirm tamponade. A typical sign of lack of "sliding" between the parietal and visceral pleura at anterior chest level has been credited with diagnostic accuracy.[10-12] So, the diagnosis of pneumothorax using targeted emergent echocardiography is based on

- Clinical suspicion
- Ruled-out tamponade
- Negative "sliding" sign

All the above-listed pathologies are essentially echocardiographic diagnoses which can be instantly recognized by a quick, two-dimensional echo scan only. The diagnostic thus obtained can immediately redirect the resuscitation effort and make the difference between a failed and a successful resuscitation.

Current resuscitation guidelines emphasize the need for recognition of the underlying pathology and correctable conditions but offer no practical suggestion on how to achieve this.[13] This reflects a recognition of the lack of availability of emergency echocardiographic imaging "in the field," though this should be less of a limiting factor in a hospital setting. Another potential limiting factor is the concern with the possible interruptions and delay introduced by echo imaging in the CPR sequence. However, echo scanning needs not to interfere with the resuscitative manoeuvres as it can be performed with very brief interruptions during cardiac compressions, from a subcostal or apical window. *Since only a reasonable quality two-dimensional image is needed, a small, portable hand-held unit can provide vital information even in "field" conditions. Alternatively, in a hospital setting, in already intubated patients, emergency TEE is a practical alternative of recognized value.*[4,14]

Suspected tamponade and PEA have been long recognized as a clear indication for emergency echocardiography,[15] and in selected cases, brief scanning should be performed during resuscitation without deleterious effect on the timing and efficacy of cardiac massage or ventilation.

Prompted by case reports and the acknowledged diagnostic value of echocardiography in these situations, there is a growing recognition of the crucial role of a quick, targeted scan in the management of patients with PEA.[7–9] Protocols such as CAUSE (Cardiac Arrest Ultrasound Examination) or FEER (Focused Echocardiographic Evaluation in Resuscitation management) have been recommended to standardize an echo-based approach and each medical institution should, ideally, establish its own pathway to include echocardiography during resuscitation. *A possible algorithm for Echo-Guided Advanced Life Support (EGALS) in patients with nonshockable rhythms is suggested below* (Fig. 11.1) *and may be regarded as a variant of the Immediate Echocardiographic Triage (IMET) pathway* (Fig. 2.1) *described in Sect. 2.1.2, targeted for resuscitation scenarios.*

11.3 ECHOCARDIOGRAPHY AFTER RESUSCITATION

There are no formal guidelines for the use of echocardiography in successfully resuscitated patients after nontraumatic sudden cardiac death. In previously healthy patients and if the etiology is not clear (e.g., primary ventricular fibrillation in the setting of acute myocardial infarction), echocardiography should be strongly considered to assess for the following:

1. Conditions associated with malignant arrhythmias
   (a) Severe LV systolic dysfunction
   (b) Hypertrophic cardiomyopathy
   (c) Arrhythmogenic right ventricular cardiomyopathy

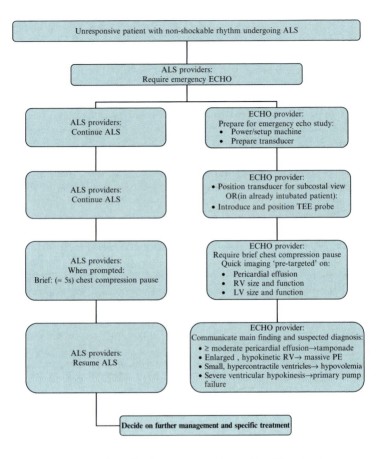

FIG. 11.1. EGALS Algorithm in patients with nonshockable rhythms.

2. Pulmonary embolism
3. Aortic dissection
4. Tamponade

Besides the possible diagnostic benefit in these patients, echocardiography may again assist with management in cases of hemodynamic instability and further risk stratification.

Caveats: shortly after resuscitation, LV contractility may be depressed due to a combination of hypoxemia, acidosis, and myocardial ischemia but has been shown to improve in a significant percentage of patients.[16] A clue to this possibility may be the lack of ventricular and atrial enlargement which generally accompany long-standing LV dysfunction but in most cases echocardiography should be repeated later to rule out postresuscitation stunning.

References

1. Memtsoudis SG, Rosenberger P, Loffler M, et al. The usefulness of transesophageal echocardiography during intraoperative cardiac arrest in noncardiac surgery. Anesth Analg 2006;102:1653–1657.
2. Redberg RF, Tucker K, Schiller NB. Transesophageal echocardiography during cardiopulmonary resuscitation. *Cardiol Clin.* 1993;11(3):529–535.
3. Lin T, Chen Y, Lu C, Wang M. Use of transoesophageal echocardiography during cardiac arrest in patients undergoing elective non-cardiac surgery. Br J Anaesth 2006;96:167–170.
4. van der Wouw PA, Koster RW, Delemarre BJ, de Vos R, Lampe-Schoenmaeckers AJ, Lie KI. Diagnostic accuracy of transesophageal echocardiography during cardiopulmonary resuscitation. J Am Coll Cardiol 1997;30:780–783.
5. Bocka JJ, Overton DT, Hauser A. Electromechanical dissociation in human beings: an echocardiographic evaluation. *Ann Emerg Med.* 1988;17(5):450–452.
6. Salen P, Melniker L, Chooljian C, et al. Does the presence or absence of sonographically identified cardiac activity predict resuscitation outcomes of cardiac arrest patients? Am J Emerg Med 2005;23:459–462.
7. Breitkreutz R, Walcher F, Seeger FH. Focused echocardiographic evaluation in resuscitation management: concept of an advanced life support-conformed algorithm. *Crit Care Med.* 2007;35(Suppl. 5):S150–S161.
8. Hernandez C, Shuler K, Hannan H, Sonyika C, Likourezos A, Marshall J. C.A.U.S.E.: Cardiac arrest ultra-sound exam--a better approach to managing patients in primary non-arrhythmogenic cardiac arrest. Resuscitation 2008;76:198–206.
9. Jones AE, Tayal VS, Sullivan DM, Kline JA. Randomized, controlled trial of immediate versus delayed goal-directed ultrasound to identify the cause of nontraumatic hypotension in emergency department patients. Crit Care Med 2004;32:1703–1708.
10. Dulchavsky SA, Schwarz KL, Kirkpatrick AW, et al. Prospective evaluation of thoracic ultrasound in the detection of pneumothorax. J Trauma 2001;50:201–205.
11. Kirkpatrick AW, Sirois M, Laupland KB, et al. Hand-held thoracic sonography for detecting post-traumatic pneumothoraces: the Extended Focused Assessment with Sonography for Trauma (EFAST). J Trauma 2004;57:288–295.
12. Knudtson JL, Dort JM, Helmer SD, Smith RS. Surgeon-performed ultrasound for pneumothorax in the trauma suite. J Trauma 2004;56:527–530.
13. Nolan JP, Deakin CD, Soar J, Bottiger BW, Smith G. European Resuscitation Council guidelines for resuscitation 2005. Section 4. Adult advanced life support. Resuscitation 2005;67 Suppl 1:S39–S86.

14. Vignon P, Mentec H, Terre S, Gastinne H, Gueret P, Lemaire F. Diagnostic accuracy and therapeutic impact of transthoracic and transesophageal echocardiography in mechanically ventilated patients in the ICU. Chest 1994;106:1829–1834.

15. Stewart WJ, Douglas PS, Sagar K, et al. Echocardiography in emergency medicine: a policy statement by the American Society of Echocardiography and the American College of Cardiology. The Task Force on Echocardiography in Emergency Medicine of the American Society of Echocardiography and the Echocardiography TPEC Committees of the American College of Cardiology. J Am Soc Echocardiogr 1999;12:82–84.

16. Laurent I, Monchi M, Chiche JD, et al. Reversible myocardial dysfunction in survivors of out-of-hospital cardiac arrest. J Am Coll Cardiol 2002;40:2110–2116.

Chapter 12
Echocardiography in Special Situations

This chapter covers complex clinical situations such as chest trauma and more focused issues including transesophageal echocardiography (TEE)-guided cardioversion, suspected stuck prosthetic valve, pacemaker optimization in decompensated cardiac failure, and mechanical support. A subsection is dedicated to the less frequent but challenging cases of acute nonischemic left ventricular systolic dysfunction, such as myocarditis or stress-related cardiomyopathies which are of special relevance to the ICU environment. The indications and input of echocardiography in the management of these challenging clinical scenarios are presented using a practical approach which makes this chapter useful to anyone directly involved in the management of critically ill patients.

12.1 ECHOCARDIOGRAPHY IN ACUTE NONISCHEMIC LV DYSFUNCTION

Coronary artery disease is the most commonly encountered etiology for the occurrence of acute LV systolic failure in clinical practice. However, not infrequently, episodes of severe acute ventricular failure are triggered by nonischemic events. This chapter specifically covers acute nonischemic conditions with documented systolic dysfunction and not cardiac failure clinical syndromes related to diastolic dysfunction, valvular heart disease, or arrhythmias. Echocardiography is crucial for proper evaluation and management in all these entities.

A. Chenzbraun, *Emergency Echocardiography*, DOI: 10.1007/978-1-84882-336-5_12,
© Springer-Verlag London Limited 2009

12.1.1 Myocarditis

Myocarditis is an acute inflammatory myocardial disease with a clinical spectrum ranging from mild ECG changes to acute onset of severe cardiac failure. It can evolve to either complete recovery or dilated cardiomyopathy. The formal diagnosis is a pathological one, however, endomyocardial biopsy is unequivocally recommended (class I) only for cases with hemodynamic compromise or associated ventricular arrhythmias or conduction disturbance.[1] Frequently, a presumptive diagnosis of myocarditis is made in the presence of otherwise unexplained acute onset of heart failure with echocardiographic evidence of systolic impairment. Echocardiographic assessment in these patients has both diagnostic and prognostic value and may also identify associated findings such as thrombi, pulmonary hypertension, or pericardial effusion.

Reported echocardiographic findings in acute myocarditis include:

- LV cavity enlargement
- LV systolic impairment
  - Global
  - Regional
- Restrictive type diastolic dysfunction
- Transient LV hypertrophy
- Increased brightness

12.1.1.1 Fulminant Versus Acute Myocarditis

Near normal LV dimensions and increased wall thickness ("pseudohypertrophy"), probably reflecting inflammatory response and interstitial edema, have been associated with the "fulminant" form of myocarditis (Fig. 12.1). These patients present with more severe hemodynamic compromise but have a better prognosis. Severe cavity enlargement and lack of transient hypertrophy are described in patients with the "acute" form of myocarditis who may have less hemodynamic deterioration on admission but poorer long-term prognosis.[2]

12.1.1.2 Acute Myocarditis Versus Acute Myocardial Infarction

LV dysfunction can be regional in myocarditis and, in the appropriate clinical context, this should not be seen as an argument against the diagnosis. Moreover, myocarditis may mimic acute myocardial infarction, presenting with ST elevation and echocardiographic evidence of regional rather than global LV systolic dysfunction.[3] The differentiation from acute MI may be impossible in the acute phase without diagnostic angiography, and this possibility should

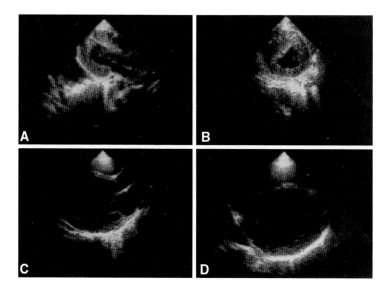

Fig. 12.1. Parasternal long (**a** and **c**) and short (**b** and **d**) transthoracic two-dimensional findings in patients with fulminant myocarditis (*upper panels*) and acute myocarditis (*lower panels*). Note the small left ventricular (*LV*) cavity size, severe wall thickening, and septal flattening consistent with pulmonary hypertension in the upper panels and the severe dilatation and remodeling with rather thin walls in the lower panels. Reproduced with permission from Felker et al.[2]

be considered in young patients with low likelihood for coronary disease, who are candidates for thrombolysis.

12.1.2   Stress-Related Cardiomyopathies

Acute, transient, LV dysfunction has been described in association with acute psychological stress or acute noncardiac illness. The involved mechanisms are not completely elucidated, but a common denominator seems to be a sudden increase in the central nervous system autonomic output. Other possible mechanisms are microvasculature dysfunction and myocardial damage mediated through a generalized inflammatory reaction. As a rule, cardiac recovery is expected beyond the acute phase and the overall prognosis is determined by the underlying disease. Echocardiographically, the LV dysfunction can be global or regional but without following the anatomical distribution of the coronary tree as in acute coronary syndromes. With some clinical entities, the echocardiographic findings are quite patognomonic, specifically involving or sparing the apex (see below).

12.1.2.1 Takotsubo Cardiomyopathy

Transient massive dyskinesis of the apex with sparing of the basal segments has been described, mainly in postmenopausal women, following an acute psychological stress, such as bereavement or a conflictual situation or in association with other acute, severe noncardiac conditions.[4] The clinical presentation, including massive ST elevation, can be undistinguishable from an acute anterior MI. Besides the appropriate clinical context, the diagnosis can be suggested by the large apical and mid-ventricle akinesis, beyond the expected damage resulting from the occlusion of one coronary artery and accompanied by a relatively modest increase only in troponin or creatine kinase (CK). A high degree of suspicion and diagnostic angiogram in the acute phase are necessary to confirm the diagnosis. The Takotsubo cardiomyopathy (TC) echocardiographic findings are detailed below (Fig. 12.2).

- Massive akinesis/dyskinesis of the apex and mid-ventricular segments (apical ballooning)
- Hypercontractile base of the heart, possibly associated with
  - Systolic anterior motion of the mitral valve (SAM) with left ventricular outflow tract (LVOT) obstruction and severe posteriorly oriented mitral regurgitation (MR)*

SAM, LVOT obstruction, and MR may develop with basal hypercontractility (see Sect. 6.4.4) but these features are not always present and are not mandatory for the diagnosis.

Hemodynamic instability is possible but these changes are transient and are likely to improve following the acute phase, either spontaneously or with cautious use of beta blockers and fluids if LVOT obstruction is present. Though major complications, such as ventricular rupture, have been described, normalization of LV function is expected within a few months or even earlier.

12.1.2.2 Neurogenic Stress Cardiomyopathy

This entity has been described mainly with subarachnoid hemorrhage where it is present with various degrees of severity in up to 30% of cases[5] but also following head trauma and ischemic stroke. Typical ECG changes include transient deeply inverted symmetrical T waves, QT prolongation, and ST segment depression or elevation. Echocardiographic findings include either global or regional hypokinesis, with preferential involvement of basal and mid-ventricular segments.[6] An apical, Takotsubo-like pattern is possible, but less frequent, being described in about one-third of the patients.[7]

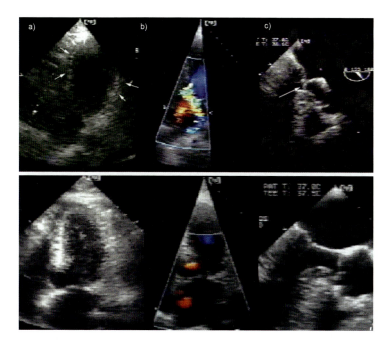

FIG. 12.2. Sequential echocardiograms in a patient admitted with cardiogenic shock and an ECG picture of extensive anterior myocardial infarction. Emergency angiogram with a view to primary percutaneous coronary intervention (*PCI*) showed normal coronary arteries and apical ballooning. *Upper panel*: echocardiogram on admission showing a large apical aneurysm (*short arrows*), severe, eccentric, posteriorly oriented mitral regurgitation (*MR*) and severe systolic anterior motion of the mitral valve (*SAM*) with left ventricular outflow tract (*LVOT*) obstruction (*long arrow*). *Lower panel*: repeat echocardiogram after 4 days shows near normal left ventricular (*LV*) function, no MR and resolution of the LVOT obstruction. **a** Transthoracic two-dimensional systolic frame in apical four-chamber view. **b** Transthoracic color-Doppler apical four-chamber view. **c** Transesophageal long-axis view of the mitral valve (*MV*) and LVOT.

12.1.2.3   LV Dysfunction in Acute Noncardiac Medical Conditions

Transient myocardial injury manifested as ECG changes, troponin release, and evidence of LV systolic dysfunction, not related to an acute coronary syndrome, have been described in patients with severe, acute medical conditions, mainly sepsis and acute pulmonary disease[6] and, generally, correlates with a worse prognosis. Evidence of non-acute coronary syndrome (ACS)-related myocardial damage was reported in one-third of the patients admitted in a medical intensive care unit (ICU).[8] Echocardiography may demonstrate global LV dysfunction[6] but some studies suggest a preponderance of anterior and apical segments involvement, with a typical Takotsubo like appearance.[9] Like for other conditions in this section, the LV function tends to normalize in survivors, after the acute event.

12.2 EMERGENCY CARDIOVERSION OF ATRIAL FIBRILLATION

Left atrial thrombi are described in 8–13% of patients with atrial fibrillation (AF) and are more likely to be present in patients with organic heart disease.[10,11] Present guidelines[12] mandate that elective chemical or electrical cardioversion of either AF or flutter of more than 48-h duration should be preceded by at least 3 weeks of anticoagulation in order to reduce the risk of postcardioversion thromboembolism to ≈ 1% as opposed to up to 7% in the preanticoagulation era.[13] In selected instances, patients with critical on-going ischemia or cardiac failure, thought to be secondary to uncontrollable AF, may be cardioverted as an emergency procedure even without prior anticoagulation[12] since the immediate benefits obviously outweigh the risks. A less straightforward scenario exists when AF is difficult to control, yet the situation is not considered critical enough to cardiovert immediately taking the risks of a stroke if the patient had not been properly anticoagulated. Cardioversion in a previously not anticoagulated patient after a TEE ruled out atrial and appendage thrombi, has been proved as safe as cardioversion after a 3 weeks anticoagulation period[14] in terms of thromboembolic risk. In a critical care setting, this approach, generally referred to as "TEE-guided cardioversion," can solve the dilemma of an early cardioversion in a patient without previous anticoagulation. However, *the documented lack of thrombi by TEE is a "snapshot" image valid at the time of the procedure only, which allows "skipping" the 3 weeks period of anticoagulation but does not in any way invalidate the need for anticoagulation*. The patient should be properly anticoagulated at least from the time of the study, at the time of the cardioversion and following it as well, according to accepted guidelines. A simple algorithm to manage this frequent scenario is outlined in Fig. 12.3.

12.2.1 Left Atrial and Left Atrial Appendage Thrombi: TEE Diagnosis

Left atrial thrombi are occasionally encountered, but the typical thrombus location is in the left atrial appendage due to the stagnant flow in this cul de sac cavity. TEE is credited in most

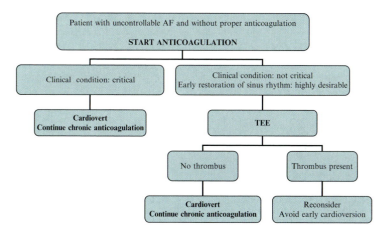

FIG. 12.3. Algorithm for transesophageal echocardiography (*TEE*)-guided cardioversion in critically ill patients.

studies with an excellent sensitivity, reaching 100%, for LAA thrombus detection.[13] This high diagnostic power requires a systematic approach. LAA is a tridimensional structure, usually multilobulated, which has to be carefully interrogated in different plans using transducer angulations of 0°, 40°–60°, and 90°–120° in mid- and high-esophageal transducer positions (see Sect. 2.2). A thrombus should be identified as a protruding or mural mass with an echogenic texture different from that of the adjacent atrial myocardium (Fig. 12.4). Differential diagnosis from an atypical LAA wall appearance or a pectineate muscle may be occasionally difficult. In borderline cases, the following findings support the diagnosis of thrombus:

- presence of the mass in more than one view
- low fibrillatory waves velocities (<20 cm/s)
- intense spontaneous contrast

In selected instances, a repeat study after anticoagulation may be necessary. As mentioned above, thrombi may form in the left atrium (LA) cavity as well, so careful scanning of the LA, using standard views and a left-to-right scanning at 0° in mid-esophageal position should be a part of the study. Also, though most reports deal with presence of thrombi in the LA or atrial appendage, the right atrium should also be scanned for thrombi as well.

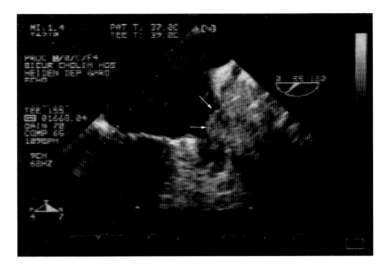

FIG. 12.4. Left atrial appendage (*LAA*) thrombus in a patient with chronic atrial fibrillation (*AF*). The thrombus is visualized as a protruding, slightly rounded mass with irregular surface (*arrows*) and a small mobile component at its lower pole. Moderate spontaneous echocontrast was also apparent in the LAA cavity.

12.3 ECHOCARDIOGRAPHY IN SUSPECTED STUCK PROSTHETIC VALVE (SEE ALSO SECT. 5.5)

Either acute hemodynamic deterioration or progressive development of otherwise unexplained cardiac failure in a patient with a mechanical valve should raise the suspicion of an obstructed or stuck valve. An alternative presentation, of stroke or peripheral embolism, but without hemodynamic compromise, should also be investigated for nonobstructive valve thrombosis. Florid endocarditis with large vegetations is another possible etiology (Fig. 12.5).

12.3.1 Questions to be Answered in an Echo-Based Approach to the Patient with Clinical Suspicion of Stuck Valve (Fig. 12.6)

- Is there hemodynamic evidence of obstruction?
  - This is, generally, a transthoracic echo assessment, so it should not be postponed until TEE is performed.

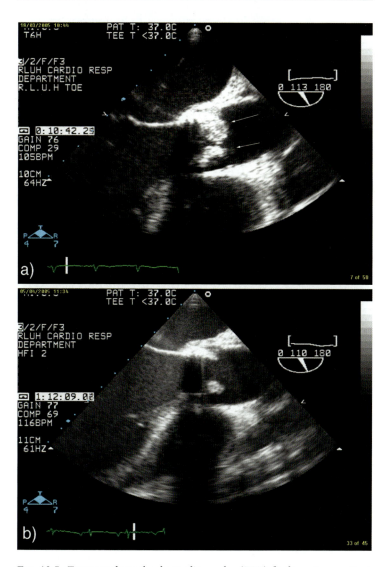

FIG. 12.5. Transesophageal echocardiography (*TEE*) findings in a patient with fungal endocarditis on a bioprosthetic aortic valve. **a** On admission: two large vegetations are present on the aortic valve leaflets, which are severely restricted in their opening motion. **b** After antifungal treatment: disappearance of the vegetations and free opening of the aortic leaflets.

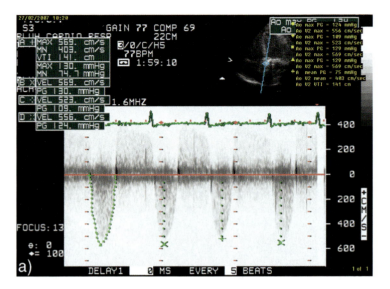

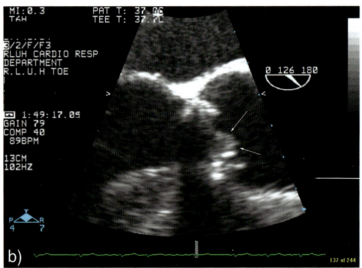

FIG. 12.6. Echocardiographic and fluoroscopic findings in a patient with obstructed mechanical aortic valve. The diagnostic sequence in this case was: TTE→fluoroscopy→TEE. Transthoracic echocardiography (*TTE*) continuous Doppler interrogation showing high peak and mean aortic transvalvular gradient systolic fluoroscopy frame. Note that the two leaflets (*arrows*), which should have been parallel to each other, are stuck in partially opened position. Transesophageal echocardiography (*TEE*) imaging of the aortic valve in long-axis view. The prosthetic valve and its motion were suboptimally visualized but a clear soft echogenic mass (*arrows*) consistent with thrombus was demonstrated attached to the valve.

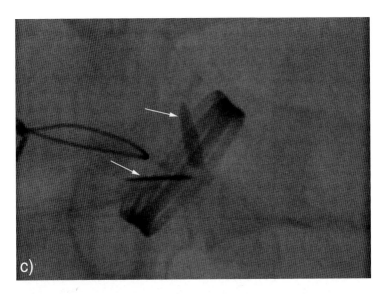

FIG. 12.6. (continued)

- o A Doppler peak and mean gradient above the accepted range for the particular valve type and size support the diagnosis of obstruction. The gradient measurement should be completed by a pressure half-time measurement in mitral position and, ideally, a calculated effective orifice area or a dimensionless index in aortic position.
- • Caveats:
  - o A significant raise in gradients as compared with baseline values (if known) may have more diagnostic information value than absolute numbers.
  - o Hyperdynamic states, such as sepsis or anemia, can raise the transvalvular gradients in the absence of obstruction.
  - o Even with obstructed valves, gradients can be spuriously low in patients presenting with shock.
- • Is there imaging evidence of reduced valve motion?
  - o This is usually a TEE assessment.
  - o Mitral prostheses motion can be generally well evaluated; however, even TEE can be unsatisfactory for aortic prostheses.

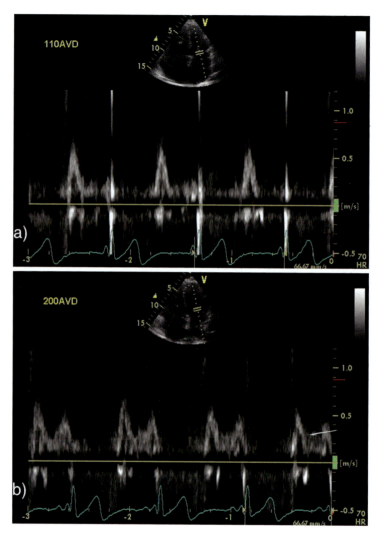

FIG. 12.7. Effect of increasing the atrio-ventricular delay (AVD) in a patient with biventricular pacemaker. **a** AVD = 110 ms: totally truncated A wave, short diastolic filling time. **b** AVD = 200 ms: full deployment of A wave with significant increase in the diastolic filling time

- ○ Practical tip:
  - □ If restricted motion is not convincingly demonstrated by echocardiography, fluoroscopy is an excellent imaging aid to assess the occluder opening and closure excursion.

- Is the obstruction due to thrombus, pannus, or vegetation?
  - Thrombus formation is a much more frequent (90%) etiology of valve obstruction than isolated pannus build up (10%).[15] With the advent of fibrinolysis as an alternative therapeutic approach for obstructed prosthetic valves, differentiating a thrombus from pannus has clear practical implications. The following clinical and echocardiographic findings support the diagnosis of thrombus over pannus[16]:
    - Shorter period from symptoms onset
    - Evidence of inadequate anticoagulation
    - Larger and softer masses by echocardiography
    - None of the above is an absolute criterion, however, for practical purposes, an obstructing mass on a mechanical valve, in the setup of poor anticoagulation status and without clear evidence of endocarditis should be considered to be a thrombus.
    - A large, mobile thrombus is considered a contraindication to thrombolysis due to the risk of embolic complications.

12.3.2 Management of Stuck Valve[17,18]

Beyond immediate restoration of adequate anticoagulation with heparin, valve replacement is the approach of choice in unstable patients without prohibitive comorbidities. Surgery is also preferred in nonobstructive thrombosed valves with large (>10 mm) thrombi or which do not respond to anticoagulation as demonstrated by serial echocardiographic evaluation. Thrombolysis should be considered as an accepted alternative to surgery in:

- Unstable patients with poor general operative risk
- Lack of appropriate surgical facilities
- Prosthetic tricuspid or pulmonary valves thrombosis.

12.4 PACEMAKER OPTIMIZATION IN THE CRITICALLY ILL

Patients with clinical heart failure, left ventricular ejection fraction (LVEF) <35% and QRS width >120 ms are candidates for cardiac resynchronization therapy with biventricular pacemakers.[19] As the use of these devices increases, so does the likelihood of being faced with patients with severe decompensated heart failure requiring inotropic support and intensive care or high-dependency unit setup, who have a biventricular pacemaker. Generally, biventricular pacemakers are programmed at default atrio-ventricular (100–120 ms) and LV–RV delays and optimization of these parameters is not routinely performed. There are no data on the impact of optimizing biventricular pacemakers in patients with cardiac failure decompensation. However, the acute changes in loading conditions and heart rate may warrant an echocardiographic interrogation to check whether the default pacemaker settings still provide the optimal hemodynamic support in the new conditions. There are two components to an echocardiographic optimization of a biventricular pacemaker:

• Pulsed-wave Doppler interrogation at mitral valve level is used to establish the mitral filling pattern and to find the optimal atrio-ventricular delay (AVD).
• Continuous wave Doppler at aortic level is used to obtain a velocity–time integral (VTI) of the aortic flow as a surrogate for cardiac output to choose the best interventricular delay.

12.4.1   AV Delay Optimization

An optimal AVD allows good diastolic filling with completion of the A wave before the beginning of the ventricular systole. A too short AVD will result in a truncated or even absent A wave, while a too long AVD will result in merging of the E and A waves and, possibly, diastolic MR. Algorithms exist to determine the optimal atrio-ventricular delay,[20] but a simpler approach is an iterative one where 10–20 ms steps are used to gradually increase the AVD if the A wave is truncated or to decrease it if there is E and A waves fusion, until an optimal pattern is obtained (Fig. 12.5). Recent data and recommendations suggest that only patients with fused E and A waves or truncated A wave need echoguided optimization of their atrio-ventricular delays.[21,22]

12.4.2   Interventricular Optimization

There are little data on the benefits of optimization of the LV–RV delay. The reported techniques use the VTI of the aortic flow, obtained with CW Doppler in the apical five-chamber view, as a surrogate for cardiac output. The measurement is obtained at nominal values and then at different LV-RV delays. The LV is generally brought forward using steps of 10–20 ms until the largest VTI is achieved.

12.5   ECHOCARDIOGRAPHY IN THE MANAGEMENT OF PATIENTS WITH MECHANICAL CARDIAC SUPPORT

12.5.1   Intraaortic Balloon Pump

The abrupt deflation of the intraaortic balloon pump (IABP) in systole and its inflation in diastole have the beneficial effects to lower the systolic aortic impedance and thus to augment the antegrade stroke volume and to increase the diastolic aortic pressure and, consequently, enhance coronary perfusion. IABP is inserted in the following scenarios:

- Severe LV systolic dysfunction due to ischemia or myocarditis, when contractility is expected to recover
- Acute MR or acute interventricular septum rupture as a bridging procedure to surgery
- Ongoing ischemia as a bridge to revascularization
- As a supportive measure following selected percutaneous coronary interventions

Essential uses of transthoracic echocardiography (TTE) in patients considered for IABP:

- Confirm and refine the diagnosis
- Rule out significant aortic regurgitation which is a contraindication to IABP

Possible roles of TEE in patients considered for IABP or with an IABP in situ:

- Rule out descending aortic aneurysm or severe atherosclerosis with complex plaques and/or mobile atheroma (Fig. 2.8b)
- Assist with placement of the balloon:
  - The tip of the balloon should be visualized a few centimeters below the origin of the left subclavian artery
  - Advancing and withdrawing the balloon under TEE monitoring may obviate the need for multiple X-rays studies
- Confirm proper inflation and deflation of the balloon
- Monitor LV systolic improvement or decrease of regurgitant flow with acute MR (TTE or TEE).

12.5.2   Left Ventricular Assist Device

Left ventricular assist devices (LVAD) may be used in patients with end-stage cardiac failure as a bridging procedure to heart transplant. Blood is suctioned into the pump through a unidirectional valved conduit inserted in the LV apex and is expelled through a second valved conduit into the ascending aorta. As a result, there is marked unloading of the left heart, which may be critical if significant aortic regurgitation or a patent foramen ovale (PFO) are present. Also, satisfactory RV function is essential to ensure adequate return to the left ventricle. Echocardiography is mandatory in the preoperative assessment of these patients and is extensively used during and immediately after the procedure and for long-term monitoring of complications as well.[23,24] The following is a list of pathologies to be specifically sought as part of a comprehensive preimplantation echocardiographic evaluation[24]:

- PFO
- Aortic regurgitation
- RV function
- LV, LA, or LAA thrombus

12.6 ECHOCARDIOGRAPHY IN THE ASSESSMENT OF TRAUMA PATIENT

Echocardiographic evaluation in trauma patients may be immediately targeted to suspected heart or great vessels injuries or included as part of a comprehensive ultrasound assessment of multiple traumas even in the absence of clear evidence for cardiac involvement. The need and focus of echocardiographic assessment in a trauma patient are dictated by:

- The site(s) of the injury
  - Chest
  - Abdomen
- The hemodynamic status
  - Stable
  - Unstable
- Evidence of cardiac and/or great vessels injury
  - Identified penetrating or blunt chest injury
  - Pathological murmurs
  - Abnormal ECG
  - Arrhythmias
  - Rise in cardiac biochemical markers
  - Abnormal chest X-ray
  - Cardiomegaly
  - Widened mediastinum

The technique involved may vary from a quick subcostal scan with a hand-held machine to rule out tamponade to a full TEE study for suspected aortic rupture. The role of echocardiography in chest and abdominal trauma is discussed below; however, in real life scenarios of polytrauma patients, this classification may be oversimplistic and an integrated approach is essential. Ideally, these patients should be managed in trauma centers, but all institutions need to have an algorithm in place defining the indications for emergency echocardiography in trauma patients, its role as opposed to other imaging or exploratory techniques and when a formal cardiology consultation is required. Since sonographers or cardiologists are not always immediately available, the need for training of emergency and trauma doctors in performing simple and focused ultrasound studies is increasingly recognized.[25]

12.6.1   Penetrating Chest Trauma

Patients with obvious penetrating chest injuries presenting with shock or moribund, are generally not candidates for immediate imaging studies and are triaged for fluid resuscitation and instant exploratory surgery. Hemodynamically stable victims of penetrating chest injuries may still have occult cardiac lesions, leading to slow or delayed development of tamponade. Two-dimensional echocardiography is a quick, accurate, readily available, and easy to repeat test to confirm or rule out progressive accumulation of pericardial fluid. Some authors report a low sensitivity of TTE for occult cardiac injuries in the presence of hemothorax, possibly due to continuous self-drainage of the pericardial fluid into the pleural space.[26] However, in most studies, TTE compared favorably with subxyphoid pericardial window (SPW) in the diagnosis of occult cardiac injuries. Since SPW is an invasive surgical technique with a high negative yield rate, TTE screening, alone or combined with chest computed tomography (CT), is advocated as a noninvasive alternative for evaluation and monitoring of stable patients with penetrating chest injuries.[27,28]

12.6.2   Blunt Chest Trauma

Damage to both the heart and the great vessels can occur in nonpenetrating chest injury (Fig. 12.8) with an estimated incidence of 15% and 4%, respectively, in series of patients with blunt chest trauma.[29] A lack of obvious chest wall lesions makes cardiac injury less likely but does not rule it out. Hemodynamic instability should raise the suspicion of cardiac injury; however, polytrauma patients may have noncardiac causes of hemodynamic instability as well, such as bleeding, spinal shock, or pneumothorax, so a multipronged assessment strategy is essential. The main mechanisms involved in blunt heart trauma are heart compression between the sternum and the thoracic spine, direct damage by a fractured sternum, and deceleration or traction/torsion injuries.

12.6.3   Cardiac Contusion

Cardiac contusion represents the most frequently encountered injury in patients with blunt chest trauma. The RV is more commonly involved than the LV. Pathologically, cardiac contusion results in necrotic and hemorrhagic ventricular areas leading to ventricular dysfunction. The clinical picture varies from pain only, which may be difficult to differentiate from chest wall trauma-related symptoms, to ECG changes, arrhythmias, and pump failure. Mild cases generally have a good prognosis.

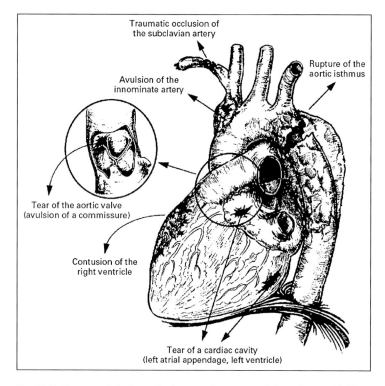

FIG. 12.8. Common injuries to the heart and great vessels in patients with blunt chest trauma. Reproduced with permission from Pretre and Chilcott.[29]

Echocardiographic findings in isolated cardiac contusion include segmental wall motion abnormalities and ventricular enlargement. *Any other valvular lesions, pericardial effusion or great vessels injury should also be actively sought*. As a readily available and noninvasive test, echocardiography should be liberally used in chest trauma victims; however, it has been shown to have a limited screening value in patients without any clinical suspicion of cardiac involvement. Moreover, TTE studies may be impractical due to chest wall lesions or tenderness; TEE is safe, though caution is necessary in the presence of spinal injury and should not be used as a screening technique in the absence of a clear indication. Routine echocardiographic imaging for cardiac contusion is thus not necessary in most stable patients with mild chest trauma and normal ECG and chest radiography.[27,30] The following are considered to represent indications for echocardiographic evaluation in blunt chest trauma:

- Cardiac sounding chest pain or dyspnea
- Hemodynamic instability
- Abnormal chest X-ray
- Severe chest trauma with sternal fracture
- Raised troponin levels
- New onset arrhythmias
- ECG changes

12.6.4 Valvular Lesions and Ventricular Wall Laceration

An abrupt rise in intracavitary pressure due to extreme cardiac compression may induce valvular disruptions, coronary injury, or even ventricular wall rupture or dissection. Though they represent advanced forms of cardiac contusion, they are generally dealt with as separate entities. Many of these patients present with extreme hemodynamic compromise but late-developing tamponade or valve failure have been reported. A high degree of suspicion is thus necessary and echocardiography should be used in severe chest trauma even in the absence of obvious cardiac involvement at the time of presentation.

12.6.5 Great Vessels Trauma

Early data underline the possible catastrophic outcome of traumatic aortic injury, with only one-fifth of the patients surviving long enough to reach a hospital.[31] The descending aorta can be injured, mainly at isthmus level, in horizontal deceleration injuries such as in a car crash. The ascending aorta can be injured in vertical deceleration accidents such as high height falls and the arch vessels can be damaged by sudden neck extension.[29,30] The resultant lesions may vary from intimal tears and dissection to medial disruption with intramural hematoma or full rupture. A high degree of diagnostic suspicion is necessary in survivors of high-speed deceleration-type accidents even if clinical evidence of chest trauma or aortic injury is not obvious on admission since specific signs or symptoms may be absent in more than 50% of cases.[30] Chest radiography is a valuable screening test; however, its specificity is low and the sensitivity is not good enough to rule out traumatic aortic pathology when clinical suspicion is high. The main contenders for noninvasive assessment of these patients are helical CT and TEE, both reported to have a predictive value of 100%.[30] TEE findings in traumatic aortic injury include thick intraluminal stripes, intimal flaps, wall hematomas, and aneurysms and pseudoaneurysms.[32] The presence of a significant mediastinal hematoma, identified as an increased distance from the transducer to the anterior aortic wall or from the posterior aortic

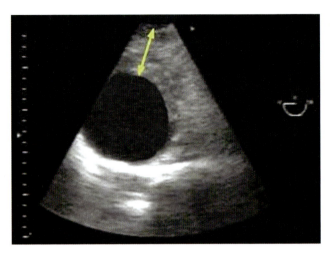

Fig. 12.9. Mediastinal periaortic hematoma in a case of descending aorta rupture. Note the increased distance from the esophagus to the anterior aortic wall (*arrows*). Reproduced with permission from Evangelista et al.[34]

wall to the left visceral pleura,[33,34] is also considered a marker for possible aortic injury even when direct findings are not demonstrated,[35] (Fig. 12.9). The distal ascending aorta and the arch are not well visualized with TEE and accuracy is dependent on operator expertise, but these limitations are counterbalanced by its immediate bedside availability and the option to be performed at the time of exploratory surgery.

12.6.6   Commotio Cordis
Ventricular fibrillation and sudden death are rarely reported in youngsters without organic heart disease, following a relatively low energy blow to the precordium, typically occurring during sport activities.[36] The mechanism seems to be induction of ventricular fibrillation by mechanical impact, typically not severe enough to result in identifiable trauma, but occurring within a vulnerable 15–30 ms time-window prior to the T wave. Successfully resuscitated survivors of suspected commotio cordis need to be thoroughly investigated, including echocardiography, to rule out both acute pathology related to chest trauma and underlying cardiac disorder.[36]

12.6.7 Abdominal Trauma

Ultrasound assessment is formally incorporated in trauma evaluation protocols during either primary or secondary survey and is reported to be used in 80% of trauma centers and to have significantly reduced the use of peritoneal lavage as a screening test in the United States.[37,38] In patients with abdominal trauma, isolated or as part of a multiple trauma case, a Focused Assessment by Sonography in Trauma (FAST) examination is used to specifically identify the presence of hemoperitoneum or tamponade. This is performed as a quick, bedside screening procedure, with a portable or hand-held machine, using the following windows[39]:

- Subcostal view: subxyphoid window
- Right upper quadrant (Morison pouch) view: left mid-axillary line, ribs 11–12 window
- Left upper quadrant view: right mid-axillary line, ribs 10–11window
- Pelvis view: suprapubic window

The diagnostic predictive value of the FAST protocol for intraabdominal injury is highest for unstable patients. Complementary studies may be necessary in stable patients, depending on clinical suspicion.[40]

References

1. Cooper LT, Baughman KL, Feldman AM, et al. The role of endomyocardial biopsy in the management of cardiovascular disease: a scientific statement from the American Heart Association, the American College of Cardiology, and the European Society of Cardiology Endorsed by the Heart Failure Society of America and the Heart Failure Association of the European Society of Cardiology. Eur Heart J 2007;28:3076–3093.
2. Felker GM, Boehmer JP, Hruban RH et al. Echocardiographic findings in fulminant and acute myocarditis. *J Am Coll Cardiol.* 2000;36(1):227–232.
3. Dec GW, Jr., Waldman H, Southern J, Fallon JT, Hutter AM Jr., Palacios I. Viral myocarditis mimicking acute myocardial infarction. *J Am Coll Cardiol.* 1992;20(1):85–89.
4. Gianni M, Dentali F, Grandi AM, Sumner G, Hiralal R, Lonn E. Apical ballooning syndrome or takotsubo cardiomyopathy: a systematic review. *Eur Heart J.* 2006;27(13):1523–1529.
5. Banki N, Kopelnik A, Tung P, et al. Prospective analysis of prevalence, distribution, and rate of recovery of left ventricular systolic dysfunction in patients with subarachnoid hemorrhage. J Neurosurg 2006;105:15–20.
6. Bybee KA, Prasad A. Stress-related cardiomyopathy syndromes. *Circulation.* 2008;118(4):397–409.
7. Lee VH, Connolly, HM, Fulgham, JR, et al. Tako-tsubo cardiomyopathy in aneurysmal subarachnoid hemorrhage: an underappreciated ventricular dysfunction. *J Neurosurg.* 2006;105(2):264–270.

8. Quenot JP, Teuff GL, Quantin C, et al. Myocardial injury in critically ill patients: relation to increased cardiac troponin I and hospital mortality. *Chest.* 2005;128(4):2758–2764.
9. Park JH, Kang SJ, Song JK, et al. Left ventricular apical ballooning due to severe physical stress in patients admitted to the medical ICU. Chest 2005;128:296–302.
10. Manning WJ, Silverman DI, Gordon SP, Krumholz HM, Douglas PS. Cardioversion from atrial fibrillation without prolonged anticoagulation with use of transesophageal echocardiography to exclude the presence of atrial thrombi. N Engl J Med 1993;328:750–755.
11. Mazouz B, Keren A, Chenzbraun A. Age alone is not a risk factor for left atrial thrombus in atrial fibrillation. *Heart.* 2008;94(2):197–199.
12. Fuster V, Ryden LE, Cannom DS, et al. ACC/AHA/ESC 2006 Guidelines for the Management of Patients with Atrial Fibrillation: a report of the American College of Cardiology/American Heart Association Task Force on Practice Guidelines and the European Society of Cardiology Committee for Practice Guidelines (Writing Committee to Revise the 2001 Guidelines for the Management of Patients With Atrial Fibrillation): developed in collaboration with the European Heart Rhythm Association and the Heart Rhythm Society. Circulation 2006;114:e257–354.
13. Silverman DI, Manning WJ. Role of echocardiography in patients undergoing elective cardioversion of atrial fibrillation. *Circulation.* 1998;98(5):479–486.
14. Klein AL, Grimm RA, Murray RD, et al. Use of transesophageal echocardiography to guide cardioversion in patients with atrial fibrillation. *N Engl J Med.* 2001;344(19):1411–1420.
15. Deviri E, Sareli P, Wisenbaugh T, Cronje SL. Obstruction of mechanical heart valve prostheses: clinical aspects and surgical management. *J Am Coll Cardiol.* 1991;17(3):646–650.
16. Barbetseas J, Nagueh SF, Pitsavos C, Toutouzas PK, Quiñones MA, Zoghbi WA. Differentiating thrombus from pannus formation in obstructed mechanical prosthetic valves: an evaluation of clinical, transthoracic and transesophageal echocardiographic parameters. *J Am Coll Cardiol.* 1998;32(5):1410–1417.
17. Vahanian A, Baumgartner H, Bax J, et al. Guidelines on the management of valvular heart disease: the Task Force on the Management of Valvular Heart Disease of the European Society of Cardiology. *Eur Heart J.* 2007;28(2):230–268.
18. Lengyel M, Fuster V, Keltai M, et al. Guidelines for management of left-sided prosthetic valve thrombosis: a role for thrombolytic therapy. Consensus Conference on Prosthetic Valve Thrombosis. *J Am Coll Cardiol.* 1997;30(6):1521–1526.
19. Hunt SA, Abraham WT, Chin MH, et al. ACC/AHA 2005 Guideline Update for the Diagnosis and Management of Chronic Heart Failure in the Adult: a report of the American College of Cardiology/American Heart Association Task Force on Practice Guidelines (Writing Committee to Update the 2001 Guidelines for the Evaluation and Management of Heart Failure): developed in collaboration with

the American College of Chest Physicians and the International Society for Heart and Lung Transplantation: endorsed by the Heart Rhythm Society. Circulation 2005;112:e154–235.

20. Melzer C, Borges AC, Knebel F, et al. Echocardiographic AV-interval optimization in patients with reduced left ventricular function. *Cardiovasc Ultrasound.* 2004;2:30.

21. Gorcsan J, 3rd, Abraham T, Agler DA, et al. Echocardiography for cardiac resynchronization therapy: recommendations for performance and reporting--a report from the American Society of Echocardiography Dyssynchrony Writing Group endorsed by the Heart Rhythm Society. J Am Soc Echocardiogr 2008;21:191–213.

22. Kedia N, Ng K, Apperson-Hansen C, et al. Usefulness of atrioventricular delay optimization using Doppler assessment of mitral inflow in patients undergoing cardiac resynchronization therapy. Am J Cardiol 2006;98:780–785.

23. Horton SC, Khodaverdian R, Chatelain P, et al. Left ventricular assist device malfunction: an approach to diagnosis by echocardiography. *J Am Coll Cardiol.* 2005;45(9):1435–1440.

24. Scalia GM, McCarthy PM, Savage RM, Smedira NG, Thomas JD. Clinical utility of echocardiography in the management of implantable ventricular assist devices. J Am Soc Echocardiogr 2000;13:754–763.

25. Beaulieu Y. Specific skill set and goals of focused echocardiography for critical care clinicians. *Crit Care Med.* 2007;35(Suppl. 5): S144–S149.

26. Meyer DM, Jessen ME, Grayburn PA. Use of echocardiography to detect occult cardiac injury after penetrating thoracic trauma: a prospective study. *J Trauma.* 1995;39(5):902–907; discussion 907–909.

27. Chan D. Echocardiography in thoracic trauma. *Emerg Med Clin North Am.* 1998;16(1):191–207.

28. Burack JH, Kandil E, Sawas A, et al. Triage and outcome of patients with mediastinal penetrating trauma. *Ann Thorac Surg.* 2007;83(2): 377–382; discussion 382.

29. Pretre R, Chilcott M. Blunt trauma to the heart and great vessels. *N Engl J Med.* 1997;336(9):626–632.

30. Navid F, Gleason TG. Great vessel and cardiac trauma: diagnostic and management strategies. *Semin Thorac Cardiovasc Surg.* 2008;20(1):31–38.

31. Willens HJ, Kessler KM. Transesophageal echocardiography in the diagnosis of diseases of the thoracic aorta: part 1. Aortic dissection, aortic intramural hematoma, and penetrating atherosclerotic ulcer of the aorta. *Chest.* 1999;116(6):1772–1779.

32. Goarin JP, Catoire P, Jacquens Y, et al. Use of transesophageal echocardiography for diagnosis of traumatic aortic injury. *Chest.* 1997;112(1):71–80.

33. Le Bret F, Ruel P, Rosier H, Goarin JP, Riou B, Viars P. Diagnosis of traumatic mediastinal hematoma with transesophageal echocardiography. *Chest.* 1994;105(2):373–376.

34. Evangelista A, Avegliano G, Elorz C, González-Alujas T, del Castillo HG, Soler-Soler J. Transesophageal echocardiography in the diagnosis of acute aortic syndrome. *J Card Surg.* 2002;17(2):95–106.

35. Vignon P, Rambaud G, François B, Preux P-M, Lang RM, Gastinne H. Quantification of traumatic hemomediastinum using transesophageal echocardiography: impact on patient management. *Chest.* 1998;113(6):1475–1480.

36. Maron BJ, Estes NA III, Link MS. Task Force 11: commotio cordis. *J Am Coll Cardiol.* 2005;45(8):1371–1373.

37. American College of Emergency Physicians. ACEP emergency ultrasound guidelines-2001. *Ann Emerg Med.* 2001;38(4):470–481.

38. Boulanger BR, Kearney PA, Brenneman FD, Tsuei B, Ochoa J. Utilization of FAST (Focused Assessment with Sonography for Trauma) in 1999: results of a survey of North American trauma centers. Am Surg 2000;66:1049–55.

39. Bahner D, Blaivas M, Cohen HL, et al. AIUM practice guideline for the performance of the focused assessment with sonography for trauma (FAST) examination. *J Ultrasound Med.* 2008;27(2):313–318.

40. Beaulieu Y, Marik PE. Bedside ultrasonography in the ICU: part 2. *Chest.* 2005;128(3):1766–1781.

Chapter 13
Conclusion

The role and advantages of echocardiography in the immediate assessment and monitoring of unstable patients is increasingly recognized and advocated.[1–4] However, except for occasional "enthusiast" units and services in large hospitals,[5,6] the "emergency" and intensive care community have been quite slow in adopting this technique. An important reason seems to be the perception of echocardiography as being primary a cardiological discipline, and also some contradictory messages about the skills and qualifications required. A sound understanding of echocardiography is essential and is advocated by the American Society of Echocardiography and the American College of Cardiology[7] which require full echocardiographic training for those wishing to use echocardiography in critically ill patients. However, providing this kind of training for already established anesthetists and intensivists is not practical. Besides, basic diagnostic skills to recognize major, life-threatening pathologies such as tamponade, massive pulmonary embolus, severe ventricular failure, or intraperitoneal fluid can be acquired with much narrower and reduced training. Indeed, short, focused training programs are advocated for well-defined protocols such as Focused Echo Evaluation in Life Support (FEELS) and this approach is supported by national societies.[8] Assessment of volume and filling status could be also the subject of a more focused training[4] to be provided ad hoc and also as part of the educational curriculum of physicians involved in emergency care. More elaborated use of echocardiography as needed for many of the conditions discussed in this book require either a formal, full echocardiographic training of a scope

A. Chenzbraun, *Emergency Echocardiography*, DOI: 10.1007/978-1-84882-336-5_13,
© Springer-Verlag London Limited 2009

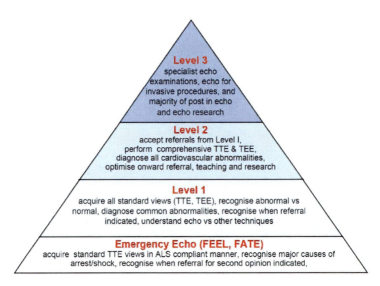

FIG 13.1 Proposed levels of competence for echocardiography in emergency and intensive care environment. (From 9, open access policy)
ALS: advanced life support, FATE: focused assessment with transthoracic echocardiography, FEEL: focused echocardiographic evaluation in life support, TEE: transesophageal echocardiography, TTE: transthoracic echocardiography

similar with that of general echocardiography accreditation, or an echocardiographic evaluation provided by an echo-trained cardiologist. A possible model of increasing competence levels (Fig. 13.1) has been recently suggested [9]. Devising institutional protocols for cooperation between emergency care physicians, intensivists, and cardiologists and solving the accreditation and educational requirements issues is probably the main hurdle before opening the way to the revolution[4] in use of echocardiography in the critically ill patients.

References
1. Beaulieu Y, Marik PE. Bedside ultrasonography in the ICU: part 2. *Chest*. 2005;128(3):1766–1781.
2. Beaulieu Y, Marik PE. Bedside ultrasonography in the ICU: part 1. *Chest*. 2005;128(2):881–895.
3. Hoffenberg JL, Smith SR, Smith RS. History of emergency and critical care ultrasound: the evolution of a new imaging paradigm. *Crit Care Med*. 2007;35(Suppl. 5):S126–S130

4. Vieillard-Baron A, Slama M, Cholley B, Janvier G, Vignon P, et al. Echocardiography in the intensive care unit: from evolution to revolution? *Intensive Care Med*. 2008;34(2):243–249

5. Breitkreutz R, Walcher F, Seeger FH. Focused echocardiographic evaluation in resuscitation management: concept of an advanced life support-conformed algorithm. *Crit Care Med*. 2007;35(Suppl. 5):S150–S161.

6. Vieillard-Baron A, Prin S, Chergui K, Dubourg O, Jardin Fet al. Hemodynamic instability in sepsis: bedside assessment by Doppler echocardiography. *Am J Respir Crit Care Med*. 2003;168(11):1270–1276

7. Stewart WJ, Douglas PS, Sagar K, et al. Echocardiography in emergency medicine: a policy statement by the American Society of Echocardiography and the American College of Cardiology. Task Force on Echocardiography in Emergency Medicine of the American Society of Echocardiography and the Echocardiography and Technology and Practice Executive Committees of the American College of Cardiology. *J Am Coll Cardiol*. 1999;33(2):586–588

8. A position statement: Echocardiography in the Critically Ill. *Journal of the Intensive Care Society*. 2008;9(2):197–198

9. Price S, Via G, Sloth E et. al. Echocardiography practice, training and accreditation in the intensive care: Document for the World Interactive Network Focused on Critical Ultrasound. *Cardiovascular Ultrasound*. 2008:6–49

Appendix A
Basic General Formulas in Echocardiography

The formulas below are listed to provide an understanding of basic echocardiographic calculations. They are included in the echocardiographic machine software, so the operator does not need to actually use them but an understanding of the principles involved is necessary to be aware of the indications and limitations of their use.

STROKE VOLUME (SV)[1]

$$SV = \pi \left(\frac{LVOTd^2}{2} \right) \times VTI$$

The stroke volume is calculated as the product of the velocity time integral (VTI) of the flow signal obtained with pulsed wave (PW) Doppler at a given site and the cross-sectional area (CSA) of the same site obtained from the diameter measured by in mid-systole two-dimensional echocardiography. Usually, the CSA is measured at left ventricular outflow tract (LVOT) site in parasternal long-axis view and the Doppler interrogation is performed in the LVOT in apical 5-chamber view. The calculations are performed by the built-in software of the echocardiographic machine.

DOPPLER SHIFT[1]

$$v = \frac{c}{2f_0} \times \frac{f_d}{\cos\theta}$$

where f_0 = emitted frequency, f_d = Doppler shift, c = ultrasound velocity, v = blood flow velocity, θ = angle between the ultrasound beam and the direction of blood flow.

The difference (f_d) between the emitted US frequency and the frequency of the US reflected by the red blood cells is used to obtain the blood flow velocity. Though angle correction is possible, Doppler measurements are not considered reliable at $\theta > 20°$.

CONTINUITY EQUATION[2]

This approach assumes that flow at two cardiac sites must be the same in the absence of regurgitation or shunt. Accordingly, the measurable flow at one site, using CSA and VTI can be used to calculate the effective area at a different site where only the VTI is measurable. The continuity equation can be used for any valve, but most frequently the flow at LVOT level is used to calculate the effective area of a stenotic aortic valve:

$$AVA = \frac{\pi \times (LVOT / 2)^2 \times V_1}{V_2}$$

where V_1 = subvalvular (LVOT) velocity, V_2 = valvular (aortic) velocity.

The use of LVOT and aortic VTIs rather than peak velocities is theoretically more accurate, but peak velocities are frequently used with good results. The software of most machines will generate results by both methods.

THE SIMPLIFIED BERNOULLI EQUATION[1]

Flow velocities measured by Doppler proximally to- and at the site of an obstruction are used to calculate the pressure gradient across the obstruction. The gradients are part of the evaluation of stenotic valves. A simplified formula, which takes into account convective acceleration only and ignores small drops related to friction, is used for clinical echocardiographic applications.

$$\Delta P(mmHg) = 4(V_2^2 - V_1^2)$$

where V_2 = distal velocity (m/s), V_1 = proximal velocity (m/s). V_1 can be ignored at values < 1 m/s.

PRESSURE HALF TIME

$P_{1/2}T$ represents the time needed for the pressure gradient of the flow across a relatively stenotic orifice to decrease to half of its initial value. It is determined directly by the echocardiography machine from the tracing of the deceleration slope, starting from its beginning. An empirically derived constant relates the $P_{1/2}T$ of the diastolic mitral flow to effective area of the valve in mitral stenosis.

$$\text{MVA}\,(\text{cm}^2) = \frac{220}{P_{1/2}T(\text{ms})}$$

where MVA = mitral valve area.

The concept of $P_{1/2}T$ is also used as a measure of deceleration slope of the aortic diastolic flow. Short $P_{1/2}T$ (<200 ms) is associated with severe aortic regurgitation.

PEAK RIGHT VENTRICULAR SYSTOLIC PRESSURE ESTIMATION

Based on Bernoulli equation, in the presence of tricuspid regurgitation, the peak right ventricular systolic pressure (RVSP) can be calculated as

$$\text{RVSP}\,(\text{mmHg}) = 4(V_{TR\,max})^2 + \text{estimated right atrial pressure (RAP)}.$$

RAP can be estimated using the degree of inspiratory changes of the interior vena cava (IVC) (Table A.1).

In the absence of pulmonary valve stenosis the right ventricular systolic pressure (RVSP) equals the pulmonary artery pressure and is widely used to assess pulmonary hypertension. However, the method may not be reliable in the presence of most severe TR.

NONINVASIVE DETERMINATION OF LEFT VENTRICULAR END-DIASTOLIC PRESSURE USING MITRAL FLOW AND TISSUE DOPPLER[3]

$$\text{PCWP} = 1.24\left[\frac{E}{E'}\right] + 1.9$$

where E' is measured at the lateral aspect of the annulus (see Sect. 3.3).
PCWP: pulmonary capillary wedged pressure (used as surrogate for LVEDP)

TABLE A.1. Use of degree of IVC inspiratory collapse to estimate the RA pressure.

IVC collapse in inspiration (%)	Estimated RA pressure (mmHg)
>50	0–10
25–50	10–15
<25	15–20

RA right atrium

References

1. Rimington L, Angelsen B. *Doppler Ultrasound in Cardiology: Physical Principles and Clinical Applications*. 2nd ed. 1985, Philadelphia: Lea & Febiger; Beckenham: Quest [distributor]. xiii, 331pp.
2. Otto CM, Pearlman AS, Gardner CL, Kraft CD, Fujioka MC. Simplification of the Doppler continuity equation for calculating stenotic aortic valve area. J Am Soc Echocardiogr 1988;1:155–157.
3. Nagueh SF, Middleton KJ, Kopelen HA, Zoghbi WA, Quinones MA. Doppler tissue imaging: a noninvasive technique for evaluation of left ventricular relaxation and estimation of filling pressures. J Am Coll Cardiol 1997;30:1527–1533.

Appendix B
Quantitative Assessment of Left Ventricular Systolic Function

Qualitative assessment of the left ventricular (LV) contractility by an experienced echocardiographer is generally satisfactory for most usual clinical scenarios. Quantification of systolic function using ejection fraction may be required in follow-up studies or if needed to decide whether the patient qualifies for a given therapy or to be included in a trial. Cardiac output may be used for hemodynamic monitoring in an intensive care unit (ICU) setting. Other indexes, such as the myocardial performance index or the estimation of dp/dt, though theoretically attractive, are not of widespread use in clinical practice.

LEFT VENTRICULAR EJECTION FRACTION (LVEF)

Defined as:
- LVEF = (EDV – ESV)/EDV, where EDV = end-diastolic volume and ESV = end-systolic volume

Normal values and accepted values for decreased ejection fraction:[1]

- Normal: ≥55%
- Mildly ↓ : 45%–54%
- Moderately ↓ : 30%–44%
- Severely ↓ : <30%

The use of either M-mode or two-dimensional linear dimensions (end-diastolic and end-systolic diameters) of LV to calculate left ventricular ejection fraction is reasonable in the absence of regional wall motion abnormalities but is still subjected to errors due to geometrical assumptions about the shape of the LV.

Accordingly, the use of these methods is discouraged and the currently recommended method of choice is the biplane method of disks (modified Simpson's method), where the LV cavity is traced at end-systole and end-diastole in apical 4- and 2-chamber views (Fig. B.1) and the machine built-in software provides the calculated LVEF.[1] This method is not based on geometrical assumptions but treats the LV cavity as a stack of elliptical disks. It requires good endocardial-blood interface demarcation, so it is not always practical.

CARDIAC OUTPUT (CO)

Defined as:
- SV × HR where SV = EDV – ESV. Cardiac output is generally indexed to body surface area (BSA) to obtain the cardiac index (CI)

Normal values:

- CI: 2.5–4.2 L/min/m^2

Allowing for some geometrical and hemodynamic assumptions, the stroke volume (see also Appendix A) is calculated as the product of the velocity time integral of the flow signal obtained with PW Doppler at a given site and the cross-sectional area of the same site obtained from the diameter measured by two-dimensional echocardiography (Fig. B.2).

MYOCARDIAL PERFORMANCE (TEI) INDEX

This measurement combines systolic and diastolic assessment in a dimensionless index of global LV performance. PW Doppler in the

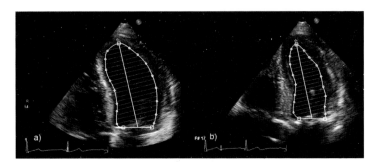

FIG. B.1: Traced LV cavity area in apical 4-chamber view for volumes and ejection fraction calculations by the echocardiographic machine incorporated software, using Simpson's method. a): end-diastolic frame. b): end-systolic frame.

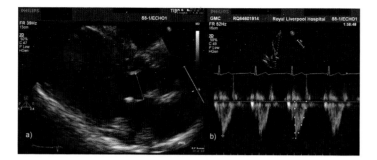

FIG. B.2: Two-dimensional and Doppler measurements for cardiac output.
a): LVOT diameter is measured in mid-systole in parasternal long-axis view between the proximal base of the septum and the anterior mitral leaflet (white thin line).
b): LVOT velocity is traced (white dots) in apical-5-chamber view using PW Doppler, with the volume sample placed at above 1.5 cm below the valve, to match the location of the 2D measurement.
LVOT: left ventricular outflow tract

apical 4-chamber view is used to obtain LV isovolumic contraction and (IVCT) relaxation (IVRT) time and aortic ejection time.

Defined as:
• Tei index = (IVCT + IVRT)/ET

Normal values:
• <0.4

REMODELING AND REVERSE REMODELING
Severe LV systolic dysfunction is frequently accompanied by remodeling, defined as increase in ventricular diastolic and systolic volumes, a more spherical shape, with a ratio >0.5 between the short and long axis of the LV and mitral valve (MV) apparatus distortion with apical tethering of the leaflets.

A reduction of ≥15% in the end-systolic volume (ESV) which can occur as result of therapy represents reverse remodeling.

LV dp/dt
The rise in the intraventricular pressure during preejection is an index of myocardial contractility, which, theoretically, is less afterload dependent. Generally measured during left heart catheterization, it can be calculated with Doppler echocardiography as well, provided that a good mitral regurgitation (MR) signal is obtained.

Using a sweep speed of 100 mm/s to improve measurements accuracy, the points of 1 and 3 m/s velocities (corresponding to a rise in pressure from 4 to 36 mmHg) are marked on the CW Doppler signal of MR in apical 4-chamber view and the time (t) between the two is measured.

LV dp/dt is calculated as

- dp/dt = 32/ Δt

Diagnostic values:

- Normal contractility: >1,200 mmHg/s

References

1. Lang RM, Bierig M, Devereux RB, et al. Recommendations for chamber quantification: a report from the American Society of Echocardiography's Guidelines and Standards Committee and the Chamber Quantification Writing Group, developed in conjunction with the European Association of Echocardiography, a branch of the European Society of Cardiology. J Am Soc Echocardiogr 2005;18:1440–1463.

Appendix C
Echocardiographic Assessment and Reporting of Left Ventricular Diastolic function

The echocardiographic assessment of diastolic dysfunction is similar to that of the filling status as detailed in Sect. 3.3. The difference is that the former is presumed to reflect the way in which the left ventricular (LV) copes with diastolic filling under steady, normovolemic conditions, while the latter is a hemodynamic assessment of filling status at the time of hemodynamic instability. If in doubt, the finding of an enlarged left atrium supports a long-standing diastolic dysfunction rather than an acute condition (Table C.1 Fig. C.1).

TABLE C.1. Echocardiographic findings in diastolic dysfunction.

	Normal DF	Diastolic Dysfunction		
		Mild (Grade 1)[a]	Moderate (Grade 2)[b]	Severe (Grade 3)[b]
E/A	>1	<1	≥1	>>1
E′	≥8 cm/s	<8 cm/s	<8 cm/s	<8 cm/s
E/E′	<8–10		>10–15	>15
Echocardiographic pattern	Normal	Abnormal relaxation	Pseudonormal	Restrictive
Hemodynamic significance				
• Relaxation	Normal	↓	↓	↓
• Ventricular compliance	Normal	Normal	↓	↓↓
• Filling pressures	Normal	Normal	↑	↑↑

[a]May be normal for age as isolated finding in an elderly subject
[b]PW Doppler assessment not reliable with severe MR

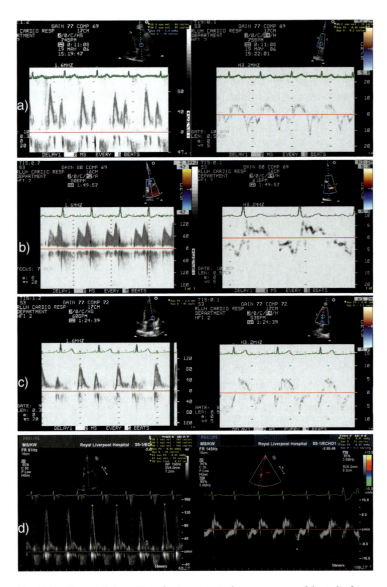

FIG. C.1. Flow and tissue Doppler imaging in the assessment of diastolic function. **a** Normal subject: $E/A = 1.43$, $E' = 13$ cm/s, $E/E' = 7.3$. **b** Elderly patient with mild (grade 1) diastolic dysfunction: $E/A = 0.8$, $E' = 3$. **c** Hypertensive patient with exertional dyspnea, normal coronary arteries, and LVEDP = 17 mm at catheterization. Echocardiography shows moderate (grade 2) diastolic dysfunction consistent with elevated diastolic pressures: $E = 95$ cm/s, $E' = 7.7$ cm/s, $E/E' = 12$. **d** Patient with severely decreased systolic function and dyspnea at rest. Echocardiography shows severe, restrictive (grade 3) diastolic dysfunction: $E/A = 4.6$, DT = 120 ms, $E' = 5.5$, $E/E' = 26$.

Appendix D
Valvular Regurgitation Quantification Principles

The true hemodynamic significance of valvular regurgitation is ideally given by the *regurgitant volume* and the *regurgitant fraction* (RF = regurgitant volume/EDV - ESV). Severe regurgitation is defined as:

- regurgitant volume ≥ 60 ml/beat
- RF ≥ 50%

These volumetric calculations are available by Doppler echocardiography, but in practice regurgitation is assessed using either surrogates related to *jet size* by color Doppler or a calculated *effective regurgitant orifice area* (EROA). The main approaches for valvular regurgitation assessment are presented below and the generally accepted cut-off values are summarized in Tables D.1 and D.2.[1] For a more detailed and in-depth discussion of this topic, the reader should consult the relevant chapters in general echocardiography textbooks and valvular heart diseases management guidelines.

- Jet size versus receiving chamber size measurements
  - For mitral regurgitation (MR)
    - Maximal regurgitant jet area/left atrium (LA) area ratio in any parasternal or apical view
  - For aortic regurgitation (AR)
    - Regurgitant jet width (RJW)/left ventricular out-flow tract (LVOT) diameter ratio (RJW/LVOT diameter) in parasternal long axis view

- Jet size at its emergence from the regurgitant orifice, *vena contracta* (VC)

  o For both MR (in parasternal long-axis view or apical views except apical two-chamber view) and AR (in parasternal or apical long-axis view)

- EROA using the proximal isovelocity surface area (PISA) (Fig. D.1)

This is a volumetric approach based on the assumption that the flow converging toward the valve on its ventricular side equals the amount going through the regurgitant orifice. The amount of blood converging toward the valve is the volume of a hemisphere defined by the plane of the valve and the aliasing boundary and which moves with a velocity equal to the Nyquist limit for that study. The EROA is given by the built-in software of the echocardiographic machine or it can be calculated as

EROA $(cm^2) = 2\pi r^2 \times V_a/V_{max}$ where r is the radius of the sphere from the valve plane to the aliasing zone, V_a is the Nyquist limit, and V_{max} is the peak velocity of the regurgitant flow by CW Doppler.

Besides the methods described above, ancillary findings have to be actively sought when significant regurgitation is suspected. These are not absolute criteria but are helpful in borderline cases.

For MR:
- LV and LA enlargement
- Hyperdynamic LV
- $E/A > 1$ with $E > 1.2$ m/s in the absence of mitral stenosis

For AR:
- LV and LA enlargement
- Short pressure half-time
- Flow reversal in descending aorta

TABLE D.1. Cut-off values for MR severity.

	MR jet area/ LA area	Vena contracta	EROA[a]	Ancillary findings
Mild	<20%	<0.3 cm	<0.2 cm^2	
Severe	>40%	>0.7 cm	>0.4 cm^2	$E > 1.2$ m/s

[a]A PISA radius of ≥0.9 cm at a Nyquist limit of 40 cm/s is indicative of severe MR. *EROA* effective regurgitant orifice area, *LA* left atrium

Table D.2. Cut-off values for AR severity.

	AR jet width/ LVOT width	Vena con- tracta	EROA[a]	Ancillary findings
Mild	<20%	<0.3 cm	<0.2 cm²	$P\frac{1}{2}T > 500$ ms
Severe	>65%	>0.6 cm	>0.3 cm²	$P\frac{1}{2}T < 200$ ms[a]
				Holodiastolic flow reversal in descending aorta

[a]A short $P\frac{1}{2}T$ is reliable only if there are no other causes of increased LV stiffness such as ischemic damage

LVOT left ventricular outflow tract, $P\frac{1}{2}T$ pressure half time

The overall assessment of regurgitant lesions should take into account more than one technique and ancillary and supportive findings as well. Jet size criteria are not accurate for very eccentric, "against the wall" jets which are assumed to be more severe than they look. Regurgitations with indices falling between the "mild" and "severe" qualifications are considered moderate

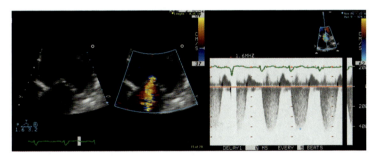

FIG. D.1 Use of PISA method in a patient with mitral regurgitation. a): The aliasing (Nyquist) limit for velocities away from the transducer is lowered to expand the convergence area and the mitral valve and the proximal regurgitant jet are zoomed-in using the apical 4-chamber view. The radius of the convergence hemisphere is measured (green dots) from the leaflets level to the aliasing boundary (bright yellow-blue interface). b): The peak velocity of the regurgitant jet is obtained with CW Doppler. (See text for calculations) PISA: proximal isovelocity surface area

CAVEATS IN THE ECHOCARDIOGRAPHIC ASSESSMENT OF VALVULAR REGURGITATION

- The color-flow display of the regurgitant jet is sensitive to the imaging settings. High gains or a low Nyquist limit can significantly increase the jet area and its turbulence pattern.

- ○ Use standard settings with a Nyquist limit of 50–60 cm/s (except for PISA calculation when it should be lowered to 40 cm/s).
- ○ When comparing two studies for follow-up purposes, ensure that both studies were performed using same or similar settings.
- Regurgitations can vary significantly with hemodynamic changes such as blood pressure, volemic status, and ventricular contractility. This may become an issue during acute or follow-up studies in the following circumstances:
  - ○ Successful diuresis and achieving normovolemic status
  - ○ Patients on dialysis who have significant volume shifts
  - ○ With improving ventricular contractility
  - ○ During transesophageal echocardiography (TEE) when blood pressure (BP) can either significantly increase due to anxiety or decrease with use of intravenous sedation (record BP during the study)

References

1. Vahanian A, Baumgartner H, Bax J et al. Guidelines on the management of valvular heart disease: The Task Force on the Management of Valvular Heart Disease of the European Society of Cardiology. *Eur Heart J.* 2007;28(2):230-268.

Appendix E

Valvular Stenosis Quantification
Principles[1]

The severity of a valvular stenosis is assessed by:

- *Mean transvalvular gradient (mmHg)*
  - Obtained with:
    - Spectral CW Doppler
  - Advantages:
    - Easy to obtain
    - Generally good correlation with stenosis severity
  - Disadvantages/precautions:
    - Influenced by the hemodynamics at the time of the study
      - Volume status
      - Heart rate
      - Left ventricular (LV) contractility
- *Stenotic orifice area (cm²)*
  - Obtained with:
    - Direct planimetry
    - Doppler calculations*
      - For aortic stenosis (AS): continuity equation
      - For mitral stenosis (MS): pressure half-time method

*For the scope of this book, only widely used methods are mentioned.

Table E.1. Cut-off values for MS severity.

	Mean gradient (mmHg)[a]	MVA (cm2)[b]
Mild	2–4	>2
Moderate	4–9	1–2
Severe	>10–15	<1

[a]In the absence of tachycardia or bradycardia, which can significantly increase or decrease, respectively, the measured gradient
[b]MVA is either measured by direct planimetry or derived using the pressure half-time method. The two methods are complimentary but planimetry, if feasible is preferable. Pressure half-time is not accurate with:
• mild MS
• >mild AR
• altered LV compliance, for example, LVH
• recent mitral valvotomy
MS: mitral stenosis
MVA: mitral valve area

Table E.2. Cut-off values for AS severity.

	Mean gradient (mmHg)	AVA (cm^2)[a]
Mild		>1.5
Moderate		1–1.5
Severe	>50[b]	<1

[a]Assuming average body-size. For large- or small-bodied individuals, the AVA should be indexed to BSA, with a cut-off value of 0.6 cm^2/m^2 BSA for severe AS
[b]Assuming normal LV contractility and cardiac output
AS: aortic stenosis
AVA: aortic valve area

Formally, valvular stenosis severity is graded using the valve area (Tables E.1 and E.2)[1].

References

1. Vahanian A., Baumgartner H, Bax J et al. Guidelines on the management of valvular heart disease: The Task Force on the Management of Valvular Heart Disease of the European Society of Cardiology. *Eur Heart J* 2007;28(2):230–268

Appendix F

Normal Ranges for Usual Echocardiographic Measurements in Adults

The values given in Table F.1 below represent a consensus of the American and European associations of echocardiography.[1] Different national bodies may adopt slightly different values.[2] Each echocardiography service needs to adopt its own standards, based on national or international recommendations and local practice.

TABLE F.1. Standard dimensions and flow velocity measurements and normal values.[1,2]

	2D/M mode	Measurements[a]
	Not-indexed	BSA indexed (/m² BSA)[b]
LVDd (cm)	3.9–5.9	2.4–3.1
Fractional shortening (%)	27–45	
IVSd (cm)	0.6–1	
LVPWd (cm)	0.6–1	
RVOT (cm)	2.5–2.9	
RV free wall thickness (cm)	0.5	
LA diameter (cm)	2.7–4	1.5–2.3
LA area (cm2)	<20	
LA volume (ml)	22–58	<29

(continued)

TABLE F.1. (continued)

| | 2D/M mode | Measurements[a] |
	Not-indexed	BSA indexed (/m² BSA)[b]
Aortic root (sinuses level) (cm)	<4	Age and BSA nomograms needed to identify dilatation
	Doppler	Peak velocities
Mitral diastolic flow (m/s)	0.6–1.3	
Tricuspid diastolic flow (m/s)	0.3–0.7	
Pulmonary flow (m/s)	0.6–0.9	
LVOT (m/s)	0.7–1.1	
Aorta (m/s)	1–1.7	

[a]Linear dimensions can be obtained by either M mode or M-mode guided two-dimensional measurements, depending on image quality and orientation. Because of technological advances, the use of the actual blood-tissue interface rather than the original leading edge-to leading edge requirement is suggested now for linear measurements

[b]For clinical use, some measurements need indexing to body surface area as emphasized above. This may be critical especially for borderline values and individuals with body size significantly below or above the average

RVOT right ventricular outflow tract, *LVOT* left ventricular outflow tract, *LA* left atrium, *RV* right ventricular, *LVD*d left ventricular diastolic dysfunction, *IVSd* interventricular septal wall thickness in diastole, *LVPWd* left ventricular posterior wall dimensions, *BSA* body surface area

References

1. Lang RM, Bierig M, Devereux RB, et al. Recommendations for chamber quantification: a report from the American Society of Echocardiography's Guidelines and Standards Committee and the Chamber Quantification Writing Group, developed in conjunction with the European Association of Echocardiography, a branch of the European Society of Cardiology. J Am Soc Echocardiogr 2005;18:1440–1463.
2. http://www.bsecho.org/Guidelines%20for%20Chamber%20Quantification.pdf

Appendix G
Echocardiographic Assessment of Prosthetic Valves

Prosthetic valve assessment may be a challenging task. Ideally, the sonographer should know the type and size of the imaged valve and be familiar with its echocardiographic appearance and normal flow characteristics (Fig. G.1). Each echocardiography service should have reference values and images of typical regurgitant flow patterns for commonly used prosthetic valves.

Besides the overall appearance and motion, the echocardiographic evaluation of a prosthetic valve will address:

REGURGITANT JETS

A trivial and up to mild degree of regurgitation is accepted for an otherwise normally functioning valve. It is seen in virtually all mechanical valves and occasionally in bioprosthetic valves. This "physiologic" regurgitation in mechanical valves is due to two mechanisms:

- a built-in-leakage which allows the valve to be "washed" by the flowing blood and
- a small amount of blood which is moved by the occluder on its way to a closing position (closure volume).

Clues for the "normal" character of regurgitation noted with a mechanical valve include:

- Low velocity, "smooth," and short (<2–3 cm) jets, though exceptions exist:
  ○ Some Medtronic-Hall valves may have a long, impressive jet

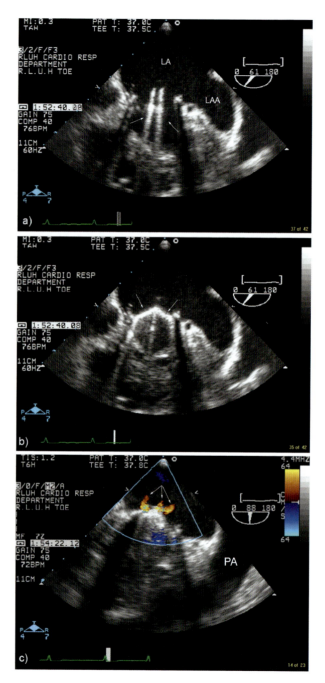

FIG. G.1. Transesophageal echocardiography (*TEE*) imaging of a normally functioning St. Jude valve in mitral position. **a** Diastolic frame showing

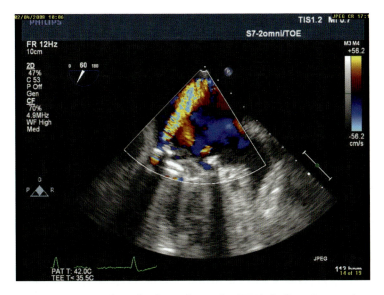

FIG. G.2. Transesophageal echocardiography (*TEE*) findings in a patient with a bileaflet mechanical valve in mitral position, admitted with cardiac failure and hemolytic anemia. A high velocity, turbulent regurgitant jet is seen, originating at the suture line level consistent with significant paravalvular regurgitation.

- Jets origin is "within the valve" as opposed to paravalvular leaks (Fig. G.2)
- The appearance of one or multiple jets with a pattern that fits the description for a particular kind of valve
  - Bileaflet valves may have up to three to four jets at the periphery of the valve (Fig. G.1c)
- Overall severity is no more than mild

PRESSURE GRADIENTS, PRESSURE HALF-TIMES AND EFFECTIVE AREAS

Pressure gradients across prosthetic valves are obtained with Doppler interrogation as for native valves and should be interpreted against published normal values.[1] Increased gradients may

FIG. G.1. (continued) symmetrical and almost parallel leaflets ensuring full opening of the valve. **b** Systolic frame confirming symmetrical and simultaneous closure of the leaflets. **c** Color-Doppler systolic frame showing three short, low-velocity jets, typical for this valve.

suggest obstruction, but some caveats are to be observed before making the diagnosis of stuck valve, especially if this is an incidental finding in an asymptomatic patient:

- Gradients may be high with small diameter valves if valve-patient mismatch exists. Ideally, a study performed in steady conditions after surgery (but not immediately postoperatively) should be available for comparison.
- Gradients may significantly increase with high output states such as acute febrile disease, dialysis patients with shunts, and hyperthyroidism. Also, mitral gradients can increase markedly with high heart rates.
- A disproportionately high-peak gradient with a minimally elevated mean gradient in a prosthetic valve in mitral position is highly suggestive of regurgitation rather than obstruction.

Dimensionless Velocity Index (DVI). Peak velocities and gradients are highly dependent on flow and their use as isolated findings to diagnose valve obstruction may be limited. With changing flows, aortic valvular and subvalvular velocities are expected to maintain their relative ratio. The left ventricular outflow tract (LVOT) peak velocity/aortic valve peak velocity ratio is referred to as the DVI. A DVI 0.25–0.3 suggests valvular stenosis.

Effective areas for prosthetic aortic valves can be calculated using continuity equation and compared with published references. For prosthetic valves in mitral position a prolonged pressure half-time value can indicate obstruction. The pressure half-time ($P_{1/2}T$) has not been thoroughly validated for prosthetic valves areas and its value should be reported as such, but resulting areas are frequently reported for practical reasons.

REFERENCE VALUES

There is a multitude of data on normal Doppler values for prosthetic valves, however, they represent a mixture of in-vitro and in-vivo, manufacturer-provided, clinical and experimental studies, some of which use only velocities or only gradients and report mean and standard deviation (SD) only or range of values as well. Also, areas and gradients vary greatly with valve size and flow state at the time of the study. As such, it is difficult to summarize the existent information.[1-2] A compilation of orientative range of accepted maximal values is provided below, to "flag" a possible pathology and to be used with detailed published data on specific prosthetic valves.

Low valvular areas and gradients at the upper limit of the range are associated with small size valves and do not necessarily mean that the valve is malfunctioning. Some valves, such as

TABLE G.1. Acceptable values for biological and mechanic porsthetic valves over available sizes range.

AORTIC POSITION		
Peak velocity range (m/s)	Mean gradient range (mm Hg)	AVA (cm^2)
1.4–4	5–30	1–3

MITRAL POSITION		
Peak velocity range (m/s)	Mean gradient range (mm Hg)	P ½ T (ms)
1.2–2	1–8	60–160

AVA: aortic valve area, P ½ T: pressure half-times

the ball-cage Starr-Edwards have gradients at the upper limit of normal range.

SUSPECT REGURGITATION IF FINDING:

- High peak gradient with minimally increased mean gradient and no other evidence of obstruction
- High velocity, turbulent regurgitant jets, not typical for the valve (Fig. F.2)

SUSPECT STENOSIS IF FINDING:

- Both peak and mean gradient are elevated above normal range
- For aortic position
  - AVA < 1 cm^2 (by continuity equation)
  - DVI < 0.3
- For mitral position
  - Pressure half-time > 200 ms

Use reference values and previous studies for comparison (Table G.1).

References
1. Rosenhek, R, Binder T, Maurer G, Baumgartner H et al. Normal values for Doppler echocardiographic assessment of heart valve prostheses. *J Am Soc Echocardiogr*. 2003;16(11):1116–1127.
2. Rimington H, Chambers JMD. *Echocardiography: A Practical Guide for Reporting*. 2nd ed. London: Informa Healthcare; 2007. vi, 148 pp.

Appendix H
General References and Recommended Reading

TEXTBOOKS
1. Hatle L, Angelsen B. *Doppler Ultrasound in Cardiology: Physical Principles and Clinical Applications*. 2nd ed. Philadelphia: Lea and Febiger; 1985.
2. Weyman AE. *Principles and Practice of Echocardiography*. 2nd ed. Philadelphia: Lea and Febiger; 1994.
3. Otto CM. *Textbook of Clinical Echocardiography*. 3rd ed. Philadelphia; London: Elsevier Saunders; 2004. xiii, 541 pp.
4. Feigenbaum H, Armstrong WF, Ryan T. Feigenbaum's echocardiography. In: Feigenbaum H, Armstrong WF, Ryan T, ed. 6th ed. Philadelphia; London: Lippincott Williams and Wilkins; 2005. xv, 790 pp.
5. Leeson P, Mitchell ARJ, Becher H. *Echocardiography. Oxford Specialist Handbooks in Cardiology*. Oxford: Oxford University Press; 2007. xxv, 549 pp.
6. Oh JK, Seward JB, Tajik AJ. *The Echo Manual*. 3rd ed. Philadelphia: Lippincott Williams & Wilkins; 2007. 431 pp.
7. Rimington H, Chambers JMD. *Echocardiography: A Practical Guide for Reporting*. 2nd ed. London: Informa Healthcare; 2007. vi, 148 pp.

GUIDELINES, STATEMENTS, POSITION PAPERS
1. Stewart WJ, Douglas PS, Sagar K, et al. Echocardiography in emergency medicine: a policy statement by the American Society of Echocardiography and the American College of Cardiology. Task Force on Echocardiography in Emergency Medicine of the American Society of Echocardiography and the Echocardiography and Technology and Practice Executive Committees of the American College of Cardiology. J Am Coll Cardiol 1999;33:586–588.

2. Lang RM, Bierig M, Devereux RB, et al. Recommendations for chamber quantification: a report from the American Society of Echocardiography's Guidelines and Standards Committee and the Chamber Quantification Writing Group, developed in conjunction with the European Association of Echocardiography, a branch of the European Society of Cardiology. J Am Soc Echocardiogr 2005;18:1440–1463.

3. Cheitlin MD, Armstrong WF, Aurigemma GP, et al. ACC/AHA/ASE 2003 guideline update for the clinical application of echocardiography: summary article: a report of the American College of Cardiology/American Heart Association Task Force on Practice Guidelines (ACC/AHA/ASE Committee to Update the 1997 Guidelines for the Clinical Application of Echocardiography). Circulation 2003;108:1146–1162.

4. Douglas PS, Khandheria B, Stainback RF, et al. ACCF/ASE/ACEP/ASNC/SCAI/SCCT/SCMR 2007 appropriateness criteria for transthoracic and transesophageal echocardiography: a report of the American College of Cardiology Foundation Quality Strategic Directions Committee Appropriateness Criteria Working Group, American Society of Echocardiography, American College of Emergency Physicians, American Society of Nuclear Cardiology, Society for Cardiovascular Angiography and Interventions, Society of Cardiovascular Computed Tomography, and the Society for Cardiovascular Magnetic Resonance. Endorsed by the American College of Chest Physicians and the Society of Critical Care Medicine. J Am Soc Echocardiogr 2007;20:787–805.

5. Lester SJ, Tajik AJ, Nishimura RA, Oh JK, Khandheria BK, Seward JB. Unlocking the mysteries of diastolic function: deciphering the Rosetta Stone 10 years later. J Am Coll Cardiol 2008;51:679–689.

6. Quinones MA, Otto CM, Stoddard M, Waggoner A, Zoghbi WA. Recommendations for quantification of Doppler echocardiography: a report from the Doppler Quantification Task Force of the Nomenclature and Standards Committee of the American Society of Echocardiography. J Am Soc Echocardiogr 2002;15:167–184.

7. Shanewise JS, Cheung AT, Aronson S, et al. ASE/SCA guidelines for performing a comprehensive intraoperative multiplane transesophageal echocardiography examination: recommendations of the American Society of Echocardiography Council for Intraoperative Echocardiography and the Society of Cardiovascular Anesthesiologists Task Force for Certification in Perioperative Transesophageal Echocardiography. J Am Soc Echocardiogr 1999;12:884–900.

8. Vahanian A, Baumgartner H, Bax J, et al. Guidelines on the management of valvular heart disease: The Task Force on the Management of Valvular Heart Disease of the European Society of Cardiology. Eur Heart J 2007;28:230–268.

9. Zoghbi WA, Enriquez-Sarano M, Foster E, et al. Recommendations for evaluation of the severity of native valvular regurgitation with two-dimensional and Doppler echocardiography. J Am Soc Echocardiogr 2003;16:777–802.

10. British Society of Echocardiography 2005: Minimum Dataset for TTE (on BSE website)

Websites

Organizations
1. American Society of Echocardiography (ASE). www.asecho.org
2. British Society of Echocardiography (BSE).www.bsecho.org
3. European Association of Echocardiography (EAE). www.escardio.org/communities/EAE/pages/welcome.aspx

Free Domain Webcasts, Images, Guides
1. ASE University. www.aseuniversity.org
2. Echo by Web. www.echobyweb.com
3. Echo in Context. www.echoincontext.mc.duke.edu
4. E-chocardiography Journal. www.2.umdnj.edu/~shindler/index.htm

Index

Printed in the United States of America